Medical Forest
Error Corrections
医林改错
Yi Lin Gai Cuo

by Wang Qingren (1768–1831)

Translated and Edited by Forest Yin

Ashi Healing Publishing

Medical Forest Error Corrections (Yi Lin Gai Cuo)

Original work by Wang Qingren (1768–1831)

First Edition: May 2025

Published by Ashi Healing

www.AshiHealing.com

Paperback ISBN: 978-1-967735-23-5

eBook ISBN: 978-1-967735-24-2

Printed in the United States of America

Medical Disclaimer:

This book is a translation of a historical medical text and is provided for educational and informational purposes only. It does not constitute medical advice or a substitute for professional healthcare. The author and publisher do not recommend self-diagnosis or self-treatment based on this work. Readers should consult a qualified healthcare professional before making any decisions related to health, treatment, or the use of herbs and formulas described herein. The content reflects historical perspectives that may not align with modern medical understanding.

Translator's Foreword

"To translate a classic is not merely to render words, but to revive understanding."

Medical Forest Error Corrections (Yi Lin Gai Cuo), written by Wang Qingren (1768–1831) in the Qing dynasty, is one of the most daring and reformist works in the history of Chinese medicine. In it, Wang challenged long-standing anatomical misconceptions, revised classical theories, and offered clear, clinically practical insights, especially in relation to blood stasis. His work is not only bold, but also deeply compassionate: it arose from frustration with ineffective treatments and a desire to relieve suffering.

Wang Qingren was one of the first figures in Chinese medical history to advocate for an anatomical understanding of the human body. Due to cultural prohibitions against dissection in traditional Chinese society, he turned to observing the bodies of those who had died from epidemics or execution. Through firsthand study and careful documentation, he constructed a more accurate understanding of internal anatomy. He firmly believed that effective treatment must be grounded in the real structure of the body, and that all medical theory should be based on practice and verification. Only then, he argued, could a doctor write without misleading future generations. In this way, Wang was not only a pioneer of Chinese anatomy, but also one of the earliest advocates of evidence-based medicine in China.

Although Wang Qingren's anatomical descriptions are now considered outdated and contain many inaccuracies— understandable given the limitations of his time—his true legacy lies in his therapeutic approach. His greatest contribution was the development of a systematic framework for addressing blood stasis and Qi deficiency, conditions he saw as fundamental to many chronic and life-threatening disorders.

Wang's emphasis on invigorating, thinning, and mobilizing blood laid the foundation for what could be called the earliest School of Blood Activation and Stasis Resolution (活血化瘀学派). His formulas for promoting circulation remain among the most effective in Chinese medicine today and continue to inform modern clinical practice. These time-tested prescriptions are preserved in this volume for readers and practitioners to study, learn, and apply.

For scholars and historians interested in the evolution of medicine, the anatomical sections in this book offer invaluable insight into the state of medical knowledge in late imperial China. Wang Qingren's writings reflect a bold attempt to ground traditional Chinese medicine in physical observation and empirical reasoning. At the same time, for readers and practitioners, the real treasure lies in his formulas and clinical discussions, which remain highly relevant for understanding and treating many conditions documented in the book involving blood stasis and deficiency.

This translation was approached not only with linguistic precision, but also with clinical understanding. As a long-time practitioner and professor of Traditional Chinese Medicine, I worked to preserve the essence of Wang Qingren's thought while presenting it in clear, accessible, and elegant English for modern readers.

This edition is designed for a wide readership: students, clinicians, historians, and anyone interested in classical Chinese medicine, especially anyone like to address blood circulation and cardiovascular issues. Where appropriate, I have preserved historical expressions and metaphors.

Wang Qingren was not just correcting anatomical "errors"— he was re-centering the role of experience, evidence, and human understanding in healing. His work remains as relevant today as it was two centuries ago. I hope this translation honors his courage and brings his insights to life for a new generation.

Forest Yin

San Francisco, 2025

Author's Foreword

This book, *Medical Forest Error Corrections*, is not intended as a comprehensive manual for treating all illnesses. Rather, it serves as a record of the viscera (internal organs). Given the observational limitations of my time, certain parts of this text may be inaccurate or incomplete. If future generations have the opportunity to directly observe the internal organs and study them closely, supplementing and correcting what I have written, it would truly be a fortunate development.

After describing the viscera, I have also included records of certain illnesses. These are not exhaustive but are meant to illustrate key patterns and principles, to help readers understand which parts of the body are affected by external pathogens and internal injuries, and how conditions of excess and deficiency present themselves in clinical practice.

If some passages seem overly simplistic, it is because medical knowledge varies greatly among practitioners. I have also deliberately repeated certain ideas throughout the book, out of concern that inattentive readers may fail to cross-reference previous sections. For instance, the chapter on hemiplegia lists forty signs of Qi deficiency, while the chapter on pediatric convulsions lists twenty. When confronted with complex or obscure conditions, one must study all sixty signs in combination, comparing them carefully to avoid diagnostic errors.

I sincerely hope that every reader will approach this book with care, diligence, and discernment.

Wang Qing-Ren @ Yu Tian

Contents

Translator's Foreword i

Author's Foreword v

Volume I 1

Preface to the Viscera Record 1

Traditional Viscera Map 13

Corrected Viscera Map 15

Record of Valves, Vessels and Chambers 19

Record of Gate, Duct, Shield and Channels 24

On Brain 29

On Qi (energy) Blood and Pulse 33

On No Blood in the Heart 39

Preface to Formulas 41

Diseases Treated by Tong Qiao Huo Xue Tang 43

Hair Loss and Alopecia 43

Eye Pain with Red Sclera 43

Rosacea 44

Long-standing Deafness 44

Vitiligo 44

Purpura 45

Purple Marks on the Face 45

Blue or Ink-dark Marks on the Face 45

Gingival Decay... 45

Bad Breath (Chronic Halitosis) 46

Women's Consumptive Disorder 46

Men's Consumptive Disorder....................................... 47

Illness Triggered by the Change of Solar Terms........ 48

Pediatric Gan Syndrome (malnutrition) 48

Tong Qiao Huo Xue Tang... 51

Jia Wei Zhi Tong Mo Yao San 53

Tong Qi San (Qi Moving Powder) 55

Diseases Treated by Xue Fu Zhu Yu Tang.................... 56

Headache 56

Chest Pain... 57

Chest Cannot Tolerate Any Pressure 57

Chest Requires Pressure to Sleep 57

Sweating at Dawn... 58

Food Travels Down the Right Side of the Chest 58

Internal Heat with Cold Exterior (Lantern Disease). 59

Depressive Stifling.. 59

Irritability During Illness 59

Excessive Dreaming at Night 60

Hiccups 60

Choking When Drinking Water 61

Insomnia 61

Infant Night Crying 61

Palpitations and Rapid Heartbeat 62

Restlessness at Night 62

Anger or Sulking 62

Retching 63

Nighttime Fever Episodes 63

Xue Fu Zhu Yu Tang 63

Diseases Treated by Ge Xia Zhu Yu Tang 66

Mass Formation 66

Pediatric Abdominal Masses 67

Fixed-Point Abdominal Pain 68

Abdominal Heaviness That Shifts During Sleep 68

Early-Morning Diarrhea (Kidney Diarrhea) 68

Chronic Diarrhea 69

Ge Xia Zhu Yu Tang 69

Volume 2 73

Preface to On Hemiplegia 73

On Hemiplegia 76

Hemiplegia Differentiation 80

Cause of Hemiplegia 82

Facial Droop Differentiation 83

Differentiating Drooling from Phlegm-Fluids 85

Differentiating Dry Stool from Wind and Fire 85

Differentiating Polyuria, Enuresis, and Incontinence 86

Differentiating Slurred Speech 87

Differentiating Jaw Clenching and Teeth Grinding .. 88

Early Signs Before Onset of the Disease 89

On Pediatric Hemiplegia 90

On Paralysis 91

Bu Yang Huan Wu Tang 92

On Plague Vomiting, Diarrhea, and Muscle Spasms 96

Jie Du Huo Xue Tang 99

Ji Jiu Hui Yang Tang 101

On Pediatric Convulsions Are Not Caused by Wind .. 104

Ke Bao Sheng Su Tang 107

On Pox is not Fetal Toxin 111

On Pox Fluid: Not a Transformation of Blood 116

On Choking When Drinking Water 117

On Itch After Seven to Eight Days of Pox 118

Tong Jing Zhu Yu Tang 120

Hui Yan Zhu Yu Tang 123

Zhi Xie Tiao Zhong Tang 125

Bao Yuan Hua Zhi Tang 128

Zhu Yang Zhi Yang Tang..........................130

Zu Wei He Rong Tang............................132

On Shao Fu Zhu Yu Tang.......................135

Shao Fu Zhu Yu Tang............................137

On Pregnancy, Labor and Retained Placenta.............. 140

Traditional Kai Gu San..........................142

Traditional Mo Jie San..........................143

Huang Qi Tao Hong Tang.......................144

Traditional Xia Yu Xue Tang....................146

Chou Hu Lu Jiu (Gourd Wine).................147

Mi Cong Zhu Dan Tang........................147

Ci Wei Pi San (Hedgehog Skin Powder)..................148

Xiao Hui Xiang Jiu (Fennel Seeds Wine)..................148

On Blood Stasis in Bi Syndrome.......................150

Shen Tong Zhu Yu Tang........................151

Nao Sha Wan (Sal Ammoniac Pill)...........154

Dian Kuang Meng Xing Tang..................155

Long Ma Zi Lai Dan............................158

Huang Qi Chi Feng Tang.......................160

Huang Qi Fang Feng Tang.....................161

Huang Qi Gan Cao Tang.......................162

Mu Er San (Wood Ear Powder)................163

Yu Long Gao 164

On Effective Formulas and Theoretical Errors 167

About the Translator.. 175

Volume I

Preface to the Viscera Record

Preface to the Viscera Record in Medical Forest Error Corrections

The ancients used to say: "If I cannot be a good prime minister, then I hope to become a good doctor." They believed that being a good doctor was easier than being a good prime minister.

I said: That is not the case. Throughout history, there have always been capable prime ministers to govern the nation. But among the physicians who authored medical texts, not one could be considered truly all-knowing. Why is that? Because the understanding of the internal organs in earlier medical texts was flawed. Later generations followed those writings and built their theories upon them, but the root of illness had already been lost.

Once the true origins of disease are obscured, then even with writing as brilliant as poetry carved in stone, or skills as refined as reshaping the heavens, the descriptions of symptoms will still not align with the actual internal organs. That is why the medical field has never produced a truly complete master.

In the practice of medicine and diagnosis, one must first understand the viscera. I have studied the theories and anatomical illustrations left by the ancients, but found them riddled with contradictions.

Take, for example, their discussion of the spleen and stomach. They claimed that the spleen belongs to the Earth element, which represents stillness and is unsuited to movement, so if the spleen moves, the body becomes unsettled. Yet later, they also wrote that the spleen moves in response to sound, and that its movement grinds against the stomach to aid digestion. If movement disturbs the body, then how can it also be essential for digestion? These conflicting statements show the flaws in their understanding of the spleen's movement and stillness.

Similarly, they described the lungs as hollow in form, like a beehive, with no open passages at the bottom, so that inhalation fills them and exhalation empties them. But then they also claimed the lungs have twenty-four openings arranged in rows, through which Qi circulates to the internal organs. These contradictions reveal similar errors in their theories about the structure and function of the lungs.

As for the kidneys, there are two, also referred to as *yao zi* ("waist seeds"). Together, they are called the kidneys, and the dynamic Qi (vital energy) between them is known as the *Ming Men* (Gate of Life). But if the *Ming Men* refers to the moving Qi between the two kidneys, then why did some also claim that the left kidney is the kidney, and the right kidney is the *Ming Men*? Since the two kidneys are a unified pair, why assign them different names? What evidence supports this distinction?

And if the moving Qi between the kidneys is the *Ming Men*, then what organ is responsible for storing that Qi? This is another example of the contradictions in their explanation of the kidneys.

Regarding the liver, they described it as having two meridians, one on the left and one on the right, essentially blood vessels. These meridians begin at the flanks, extend upward to the head and eyes, and descend through the lower abdomen, encircling the genitals, and finally ending at the big toes.

But if the liver has meridians on both sides of the body, then why did they also claim that the liver is located on the left, and that the left hypochondrium belongs to the liver? This contradiction about whether the liver pertains to one side or both reveals yet another flaw in their theory.

In their discussion of the heart, they described it as the monarch among the organs, the seat of consciousness and the source of spirit (*shen*). They claimed that intention (*yi*) resides in the heart, that intention is an expression of the heart's spiritual activity, that focused intention becomes resolve (*zhi*), that the transformation of resolve becomes thought (*si*), that using thought to plan for the future is called deliberation (*lü*), and that applying deliberation to manage affairs is called wisdom (*zhi*). All five of these mental functions, they said, are stored in the heart.

But if all of these reside in the heart, then why do they also claim that the spleen stores thought and intelligence, the kidneys govern skill, the liver manages planning, and the gallbladder controls decisiveness? According to their theory, this spiritual intelligence appears to be distributed everywhere, yet they never clearly explain which organ actually generates it, where it is stored, or how it manifests externally when it is in use. Their explanation of the heart is full of ambiguity.

They described the stomach as the organ in charge of rotting and ripening food and fluids. They also claimed that the spleen's movement grinds against the stomach to aid digestion. The upper opening of the stomach is called the *cardia*. Food and drink enter the stomach, and the refined essence is said to rise through the cardia to the spleen and lungs, from where it is distributed throughout the body via the meridians. But this explanation defies logic.

The lower opening of the stomach is known as the *pylorus*, which connects to the upper end of the small intestine. The small intestine, according to them, is the "official in charge of receiving and transforming." They stated that food and drink pass into the small intestine, transform into feces, and travel downward to the *Lan Gate* (the ileocecal valve), the lower end of the small intestine, where the clear and turbid are separated, clear water becomes urine and is sent to the bladder, while the turbid residue becomes feces, discharged through the large intestine and out the anus.

Based on this theory, urine is said to seep out from the fecal matter, so it should smell foul. But I've personally used the urine of children and spoken with those who have consumed their own urine. They consistently say it tastes salty, but does not smell foul.

Moreover, if food and water mix to become feces, then the feces should always be watery and result in diarrhea. While this might make sense for chickens and ducks, which do not urinate separately, it clearly does not apply to animals like cattle and horses that do, and certainly not to humans.

The claim that water separates from feces at the *Lan Gate* during digestion is nothing short of a thousand-year-old joke.

As for the pericardium, they offered many conflicting explanations. Some said it is the network of fine, silk-like fibers that connect the heart and lungs. Others claimed it is the yellow fat surrounding the heart. Still others described it as the yellow fat located beneath the heart, above the transverse membrane and below the vertical membrane. And then they said that the *Tan Zhong*, a structure said to have a name but no physical form, is also the pericardium.

But if the *Tan Zhong* has no physical form, then how can they also say that the meridian running through the middle finger is the Hand Jueyin Pericardium Meridian? There are so many conflicting theories about the pericardium, what exactly is it supposed to be? How can one structure have so many definitions?

The theory of the *San Jiao* (Triple Burner) is even more absurd. The *Ling Shu* (*Spiritual Pivot*) states that the Hand Shaoyin and *San Jiao* govern the upper body, while the Foot Taiyang and *San Jiao* govern the lower body, implying there are already two *San Jiao*.

In *Difficulty 31* of the *Nan Jing* (*Classic of Difficulties*), the *San Jiao* is further divided:

The Upper Burner lies above the stomach and governs the internal but not the external.

The Middle Burner is located at the middle of the stomach and controls the rotting and ripening of food and water.

The Lower Burner, below the navel, handles the separation of the clear from the turbid.

The text also says that the *San Jiao* is the pathway for the transportation of water and food, suggesting it is a tangible organ. Yet it also claims that the moving Qi between the two kidneys is the root of the San Jiao, implying that it is intangible Qi. So within a single classical text, the *San Jiao* is treated as both tangible and intangible, effectively, two contradictory concepts.

Wang Shuhe's famous line describing the *San Jiao* as "a name without a physical form" likely originated from this confusion.

Later generations proposed their own interpretations:

- Chen Wuze identified the fatty membrane below the navel as the *San Jiao*.

- Yuan Chunpu described it as the reddest internal layer of the body.

- Yu Tianmin regarded the body cavity itself as the *San Jiao*.

- Jin Yilong even proposed a theory of a "front *San Jiao*" and a "rear *San Jiao*."

The number of differing *San Jiao* theories is beyond counting on two hands. When even the most basic question, whether it is tangible or intangible, remains unsettled, how can one reasonably claim that the meridian running through the ring finger belongs to the Hand Shaoyang *San Jiao* Meridian?

Some of these theories contradict themselves; others are the misguided rebuttals of later scholars. In the end, when the foundation is flawed, every line of reasoning that follows is bound to fail.

I often had the wish to correct their mistakes, but I had no internal organs available for direct observation. I reproached myself, if one writes a book without understanding the viscera, isn't that just a fool speaking nonsense in a dream? And if one treats illness without understanding the organs, how is that any different from a blind man walking in the dark?

Though I exhausted every thought and plan, there was nothing I could do. Yet for ten years, this desire never left my mind, not even for a moment.

In the second year of the Jiaqing reign (1797), the year of *Ding Si*, I was thirty years old. In early April, I traveled to the town of Daodi in Luanzhou. At that time, an epidemic of pox and dysentery had spread among the local children. Eight or nine out of every ten infected perished. Families without financial means often wrapped the bodies in simple mats instead of coffins for burial.

According to local custom, the dead were not buried deeply. The villagers believed that allowing dogs to consume the corpses would benefit the survival of the family's next child. As a result, the graveyards were filled each day with over a hundred children's corpses, their abdomens torn open, internal organs exposed.

Each day, I passed through this area on horseback. At first, I covered my nose to avoid the stench. But then I began to reflect: the reason ancient physicians made so many errors in describing the viscera was that they had never seen them with their own eyes. So I stopped avoiding the filth. Every morning, I went to the burial grounds and carefully examined the exposed organs of the deceased children.

Among the remains left uneaten by dogs, the intestines and stomach were the most frequently preserved; the heart and liver were much less common. By comparing the remains, I found that among ten corpses, no more than three had all the internal organs intact. Over the course of ten days, I observed the full organ systems of no fewer than thirty individuals. It became clear to me that the anatomical diagrams found in medical texts did not match the reality of the human body, not in form, and not even in number.

The most critical structure was a thin membrane in the chest, like a sheet of paper, the diaphragm, essential in its function. But by the time I observed it, it had already been destroyed. I could not confirm whether it lay above or below the heart, or whether its orientation was slanted or straight. This was my greatest regret.

In June of the fourth year of the Jiaqing reign (1799), I was in Fengtian Prefecture. A 26-year-old woman from Liaoyang had gone mad and killed both her husband and father-in-law. She was sent to the provincial capital to face execution by *lingchi*, the punishment of slow slicing.

I followed the procession to the west gate of the city. But suddenly, I was struck by the thought that she was a woman, not a man, and I could not bring myself to go any closer. A short while later, the executioner passed by me, holding her heart, liver, and lungs. I examined them closely, they were just as I had seen in my previous observations.

Later, when I was in the capital, during the *Gengchen* year of the Jiaqing reign (1820), a man who had murdered his own mother was sentenced to execution by *lingchi* (slow slicing). The execution took place just south of the suspension bridge outside Chongwen Gate, and this time I was able to get close.

When I arrived, I could see the internal organs, but the diaphragm had already been damaged. Once again, I was unable to observe it in its complete form.

On May 14th of the eighth year of the Daoguang reign (1828), the rebel Zhang Ge'er was executed by *lingchi*. I arrived at the scene, but was unable to get close. I thought to myself: I am only one step away from success, so close, how could I give up now?

Unexpectedly, on the night of December 13th in the ninth year of the Daoguang reign (1829), I was invited by the Heng family of Banchang Alley, located on Andingmen Street, to treat a patient. During our conversation, I mentioned the diaphragm, something I had been focused on for forty years, yet had never been able to observe and verify clearly.

At that point, Mr. Heng Jing, Chief Secretary of Jiangning, shared that he had once been stationed in Hami and had led troops in Kashgar. There, he had seen countless corpses of executed rebels and had become especially familiar with the structure of the diaphragm.

Upon hearing this, I was overjoyed. I immediately bowed and respectfully asked him for details. Understanding my long-held frustration, Mr. Heng kindly and thoroughly described its form and structure.

I spent forty-two years seeking out and verifying the structure of the internal organs before I was finally able to confirm my findings and produce a complete anatomical chart of the viscera. I had originally intended to publish it for the world to see, but I feared that future generations, never having seen the organs for themselves, might accuse me of deliberately contradicting the medical classics.

Yet if I choose not to publish it, I worry that generations of physicians will continue to be misled, perpetuating these errors for hundreds, perhaps even thousands of years.

I reflected carefully: the Yellow Emperor, out of concern for his people's suffering from illness, often posed questions to Qibo and Gui Yuxu, which led to the compilation of *Su Wen* (*Basic Questions*). If those two truly knew the answers, then it was right for them to respond. But if they did not know with certainty, they should have waited for further study and verification. Why, then, did they give answers so carelessly, despite their uncertainty, leaving behind confusion and harm for future generations?

Later, Qin Yueren wrote the *Classic of Difficulties*, and Zhang Shixian added illustrated commentaries using the *Hetu* and *Luoshu* diagrams. He claimed that the heart, liver, and lungs could be measured in *fen* and *liang* by weight, with precise amounts for each; that the small and large intestines could be measured in *chi* and *zhang* by length; and that the stomach had a specific volume, capable of holding a certain number of *dou* or *sheng* of grain.

His statements sounded authoritative, but in truth, he had never seen the internal organs himself. He was speaking without evidence, deceiving others with fabricated details. He sought only personal fame, yet caused real harm to the world. Stealing wealth is rightly called theft, so is stealing reputation not also a kind of thievery?

How can it be possible that, even after hundreds or thousands of years, no one would see through this?

The diagrams I have drawn are not simply an expression of personal opinion, nor are they meant to pass judgment on the merits or shortcomings of the ancients. I do not seek recognition from future generations, nor do I shy away from potential criticism.

My sole wish is that those in the medical profession, upon seeing these illustrations, will feel a clear understanding arise in their minds and a brightness come to their eyes, that they may have reliable principles to follow in clinical practice, avoiding misguided paths and vague, confusing diagnoses. If these diagrams can help reduce suffering and prevent the mismanagement of disease, then my hopes will be fulfilled.

I trust that those of virtue and discernment will understand my intentions and judge me with compassion.

Wang Qingren

Written at Zhiyi Hall, Capital Residence,

Yutian County, Zhili Province

Early Winter, *Gengyin* Year of the Daoguang Reign (1830)

Traditional Viscera Map

The internal organs as depicted by the ancients appear as follows:

Lung, six lobes with two
ears, so total of eight lobes

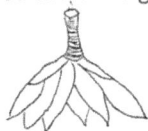

Lung

Spleen

Ileocecal valve

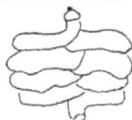

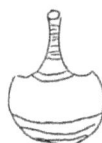

Anus

Large Intestines

Pericardium

Cardia

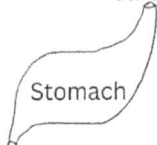

Stomach

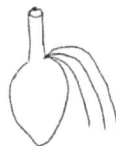

Pylorus

Heart

Medical Forest Error Corrections

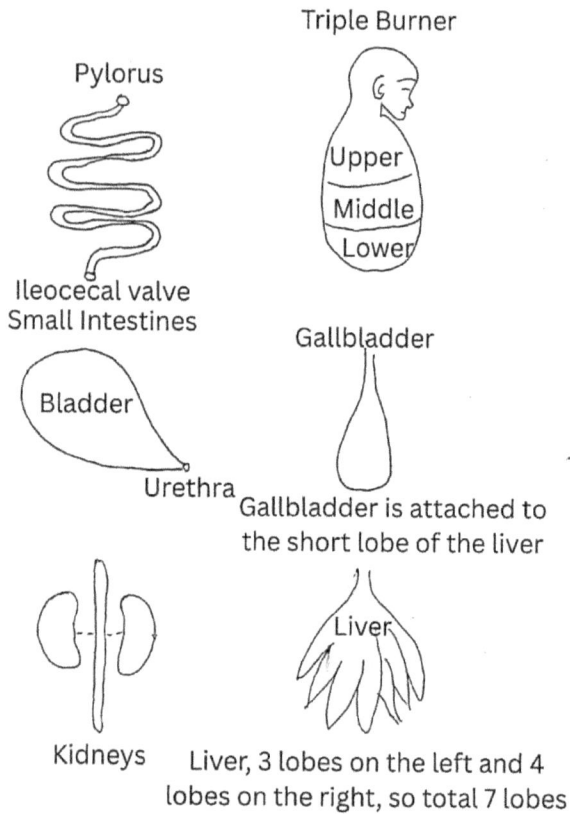

Pylorus

Triple Burner

Upper
Middle
Lower

Ileocecal valve
Small Intestines

Gallbladder

Bladder

Urethra

Gallbladder is attached to
the short lobe of the liver

Liver

Kidneys

Liver, 3 lobes on the left and 4
lobes on the right, so total 7 lobes

Corrected Viscera Map

Corrected Viscera Map Based on Direct Observation

The following are illustrations of the organs, both visible and concealed, as I have personally observed them. A total of twenty-five in all.

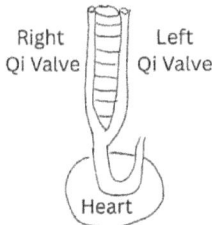

The Qi valves merge into one and enters the heart. The heart sits below the Qi pipe and connects to the Main Protective Vessel.

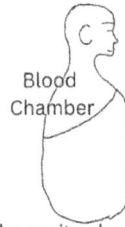

The cavity above the diaphragm, filled with blood, is called the Blood Chamber. Only the heart, lungs, and Qi valves are above the diaphragm.

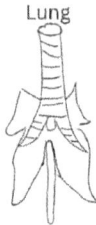

The bronchi branch through the lungs, which contain foam-like structures. The lungs are solid with no visible Qi-regulating holes.

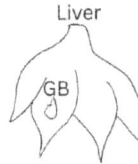

The liver has four lobes and a dense texture. The gallbladder is attached to its second right lobe, and the liver cannot store blood.

Esophagus

Fluid Duct
Pancreas
Fluid Gate
Food
Shield
Cardia
Pylorus
Stomach

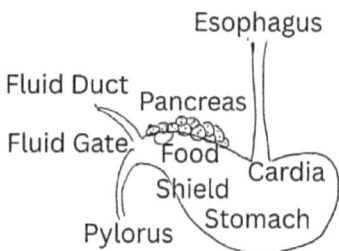

The stomach lies flat in the abdomen with its base linking to the Water Channels. To the left of the pylorus is the Fluid Gate and the internal bulge called the Food Shield. The pancreas lies to the left of the Fluid Gate.

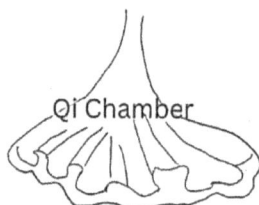

Qi Chamber

The Qi Chamber surrounds the small intestines and stores Vital Qi, which transforms food and sustains life.

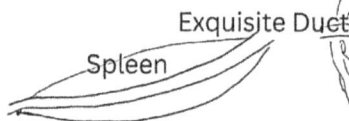

Water Channels

Exquisite Duct

Spleen

The spleen contains the Exquisite Duct, a central tube that channels water. Spleen parallels the stomach in length.

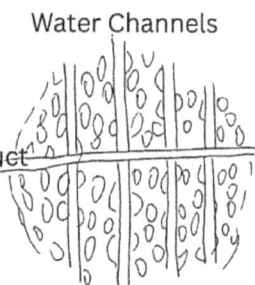

Water Channels

The Exquisite Duct runs through the center, flanked by Water Channels on both sides. Water flows through these channels and seeps downward to the bladder, eventually forming urine.

The upper opening of the large intestine is the lower opening of the small intestine, called Lan Gate (the Appendix, the Ileocecal valve).

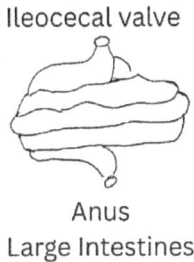

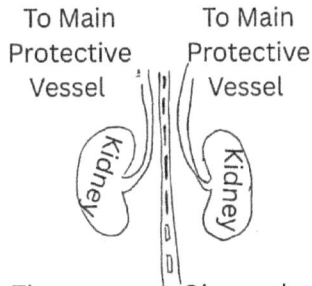

Ileocecal valve

Anus
Large Intestines

To Main
Protective
Vessel

To spine

Sperm Channel

Bladder

Urethra

The bladder has a lower opening but no upper opening, and the lower opening is into the penis. The lower opening of the sperm channel is also into the penis. The sperm channel is called the uterus in women.

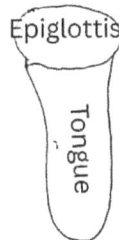

To Main
Protective
Vessel

To Main
Protective
Vessel

Kidney

Kidney

There are two Qi vessels, at the depressions of the two kidneys, connecting to the Main Protective Vessel. The kidneys on both sides are solid with no holes inside.

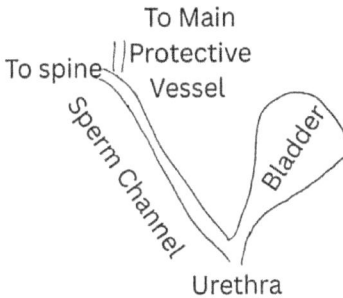

Epiglottis

Tongue

The small white piece behind the tongue is epiglottis and is the substance that covers Qi valves and the throat.

vessel coming out of the heart

Main Manifestation Vessel, Blood Vessel
Connected to Blood Residence

Left and right
to two arms

Main Protecting Vessel, the Qi Vessel—Waist-Vessel

This eleven
short tubes
connected to
Spine

Upper one to Qi
Residence
lower one to
Sperm Channel

Left and right to
two kidneys

Left and right to
two legs

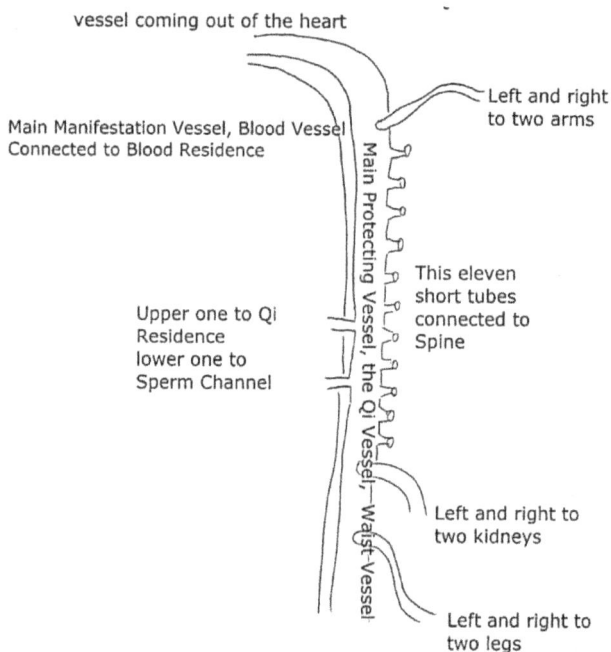

The ancients said that the meridians are blood vessels, and
each organ has two of them, but only the bladder has four. I
have seen more than one hundred viscera but did not see any
shape of blood vessels grown out of them, so write behind the
drawings as record.

Record of Valves, Vessels and Chambers

Record of the Epiglottis, Left and Right Qi Valves, General Protective Vessel, Main Nutrient Vessel, Qi Chamber, and Blood Chamber

To understand the structure of the internal organs, one must first understand the pathways of breath, both inhalation and exhalation, as well as the passage of food and drink.

The ancients said that the area behind the root of the tongue is called the *hou*, or "throat." The character *hou* also means "to wait," as it is said to "wait" for the entry and exit of breath, serving as the upper opening of the lung conduit, or trachea.

Behind the *hou* is the *yan*, or "pharynx." The word *yan* shares the same pronunciation as "to swallow", and refers to the passage through which food and drink are swallowed into the stomach. It is the upper opening of the stomach tube, or esophagus.

The claim that the *yan* receives food while the *hou* receives air has been considered a fixed truth throughout the ages. From the time of the *Ling Shu* and *Su Wen* until now, over four thousand years, no one has recognized or corrected this error.

For instance, it is widely accepted that the *yan* (pharynx) swallows food into the stomach. But the idea that the *hou* (throat) "waits" for the movement of air remains poorly understood.

They do not realize that the broad surfaces of the two lobes of the lungs face the back, with four pointed tips at the top pointing toward the chest, and a small lobe at the bottom also facing the chest. Below the trachea, the airway branches into two bronchi, each entering one of the lung lobes. Each bronchus further divides into nine medium branches, and each of those into nine smaller branches, which in turn extend into numerous bronchioles. At the ends of these bronchioles, there are no open holes or channels.

The shape of the lungs resembles *Eucheuma* (a type of seaweed), and the surface of the lungs has no openings either. The inside is filled with light, airy white foam. Contrary to traditional belief, there are no open passages at the base of the lungs, and certainly no twenty-four holes to regulate the flow of Qi.

The ancient sages claimed that inhalation fills the lungs and exhalation empties them. But these are errors that need no great debate. When air is inhaled, it is the abdomen that expands and fills, not the lungs. When air is exhaled, it is the abdomen that contracts and becomes smaller, not the lungs. Breathing in and out, coughing, vomiting, spitting, salivating, and drooling, none of these functions are directly related to the lungs.

Behind the trachea and in front of the esophagus, at the slight depressions on both the left and right sides, there are two air passages about the thickness of chopsticks. Their upper openings lie just below the epiglottis. The one on the left is called the Left Qi Valve, and the one on the right is called the Right Qi Valve. Phlegm, fluids, and saliva pass out through these passages.

The ancients mistakenly believed that conditions such as coughing, wheezing, and asthma were diseases of the lungs, simply because the symptoms appeared to come from the chest.

In clinical practice, when symptoms were diagnosed as external invasions, they were treated with dispersing herbs; when dry phlegm was present, cooling herbs were used; when there was heat accumulation, purging herbs were given; when Qi was deficient, tonics to strengthen the middle burner were prescribed; when Yin was depleted, Yin-nourishing formulas were used; and when blood stasis was observed, blood-invigorating herbs were administered.

Driven by misplaced confidence, they formulated theories and wrote books, firmly convinced that these conditions were unquestionably diseases of the lungs.

They do not realize that the two vessels, one from the Left Qi Valve and the other from the Right Qi Valve, descend along both sides of the trachea and merge into a single vessel at the midpoint in front of it, much like two branches joining into a single tree trunk. This merged vessel is about the thickness of a chopstick. It continues downward and enters the heart. From within the heart, it turns to the left and exits, about as thick as a pen tube. It travels from the heart's left side toward the back, passing to the left of the trachea, through the lungs, and reaches the front of the spine, descending all the way to the tailbone. This is known as the General Protective Vessel, commonly referred to as the waist vessel.

Below the waist, two additional vessels, also about the thickness of chopsticks, extend into the abdominal region. The upper one connects to what is known as the Qi Chamber, commonly called "chicken crown oil" due to its resemblance to an inverted cockscomb flower. The Qi Chamber surrounds the small intestine, which lies horizontally within it. The space inside the Qi Chamber but outside the small intestine is where Yuan Qi, or original vital energy, is stored.

Yuan Qi is fire, and fire is Yuan Qi. This fire is the source of human life. As food enters the small intestine from the stomach, its transformation and digestion depend entirely on the steaming and ripening action of Yuan Qi. When Yuan Qi is abundant, food is easily digested; when it is deficient, digestion becomes difficult.

What was described earlier is the upper vessel oriented toward the abdomen. As for the lower vessel, it may be connected either to the spermatic passage in men or the uterus in women. This is the only vessel I was unable to verify with certainty, despite examining it carefully. I suspect this may be its function, but I leave it to future medical practitioners, should they have the opportunity, to investigate further and provide clarification.

The General Protective Vessel has two branches, each about the thickness of a chopstick, extending from both sides of the back of the heart and growing outward toward the shoulders. At the waist, there are two vessels extending outward, connecting to the kidneys on each side. Below the waist, two more vessels descend and connect to the thighs.

Above the waist, aligned with the center of the spine, the General Protective Vessel branches into eleven vessels that connect directly to the spine. These vessels circulate both Qi (vital energy) and body fluids. When Qi is abundant and the internal fire is strong, the fluids are heated and become thick and sticky, this thickened form is called phlegm. When Qi is deficient and the fire is weak, the fluids cannot be transformed, and they remain thin and clear, this is called mucus or yin fluid.

Phlegm and mucus in these vessels are continually pushed upward by the Qi within them. They rise through the heart and pass out through the airway in front of the trachea, exiting via the Left and Right Qi Valves. Phlegm, mucus, saliva, and fluids originate in these airways, not in the lungs. The ancients misunderstood this because they were unaware that a separate airway runs in front of the trachea. Seeing that these substances emerged from the chest, they mistakenly believed they came from the lungs, simply because they had never seen the internal organs with their own eyes.

The motions of the body, clenching fists, walking, turning the head, swaying the torso, as well as daily activity, physical exertion, rest, and preservation of life, all rely on the presence of Qi. When a person inhales, the Qi Chamber fills, causing the abdomen to expand. When they exhale, the Qi Chamber empties, and the abdomen contracts.

The General Protective Vessel is the channel through which Qi circulates, it does not contain blood. If blood were to enter the Qi Chamber, it would inevitably rise or fall along with the Qi. If it moved upward, it would result in vomiting blood or nosebleeds; if downward, it would lead to blood in the urine or stool.

In front of the General Protective Vessel is a vessel of the same length and about the thickness of a chopstick. This is called the General Nutrient Vessel (*Rong Vessel*), a blood vessel that carries and stores blood. It runs parallel to the General Protective Vessel, and the blood within it is irrigated from the Blood Chamber.

The Blood Chamber refers to the diaphragm located beneath the chest. It is as thin as paper, yet among the firmest structures in the body. At the front, it aligns with the depression just below the sternum. Extending from both flanks down to the upper waist, it forms a gentle slope, higher in the front and lower in the back. The lower portion resembles a basin that stores blood, which is transformed from Essence (Jing). This area is known as the Blood Chamber. For more details on Essence, see the section below on the Stomach and the Fluid Gate.

The epiglottis, mentioned earlier, is the white flap located behind the tongue. It serves to cover the Left and Right Qi Valves as well as the throat opening (*hou men*).

Record of Gate, Duct, Shield and Channels

Record of Fluid Gate, Fluid Duct, Food Shield, General Lifter, Exquisite Duct, Water Channel

Beneath the throat lies the organ known as the *stomach* in humans. In birds, it is called the crop, and in animals, it is known as the paunch or tripe. In ancient anatomical drawings, the stomach is shown with two openings, an upper one called the cardia and a lower one called the pylorus, positioned respectively at the top and bottom of the stomach. However, what they did not realize is that the stomach actually has three openings.

The ancients drew the stomach as if it were oriented vertically, unaware that in reality, it lies horizontally in the abdomen, flat and level. The upper opening, the cardia, faces the spine, while the base of the stomach faces forward toward the abdomen. The pylorus, despite being called the lower opening, is positioned higher up, leaning toward the right flank and also oriented toward the spine.

About an inch to the left of the pylorus is a third opening, known as the Fluid Gate (Jinmen). Above this opening is a duct called the Fluid Duct (Jinguan), which serves as the pathway through which the stomach discharges refined fluids and essences. This structure is particularly difficult to observe, as it is covered by the General Lifter (Zongti), commonly known as the pancreas. The pancreas spans the right side of the cardia to the left of the pylorus, lying directly over and concealing the Fluid Gate.

The lower part of the General Lifter (commonly known as the pancreas) connects forward to the Qi Chamber and supports the small intestine, while extending backward to support the large intestine. Positioned above the stomach, it also connects to the liver behind it, which in turn is anchored to the spine. This describes the structural continuity of the General Lifter beneath the diaphragm, linking the stomach, liver, small and large intestines into one integrated system.

After food enters the stomach, the solid contents remain, while the refined essence and fluid first exit through the Fluid Gate and flow into the Fluid Duct. Just over an inch from the Fluid Gate, the duct branches into three pathways:

- The clear and light essence flows into the Marrow Chamber, where it transforms into marrow.

- The heavier, more turbid essence takes the upper branch, and, when lying down, enters the Blood Chamber, where it is converted into blood.

- The fluid portion travels through the lower branch, passes through the center of the liver, and enters the spleen.

At the center of the spleen, there is a slender, delicate duct known as the Exquisite Duct. From this duct, water fluids branch off to both sides and enter the Water Channels, whose shape resembles a fishnet, commonly referred to as "Net Fat." The fluid seeps from these channels into the bladder, where it is transformed into urine.

The process of water exiting through these channels is among the most difficult to observe. Since the second year of the Jiaqing era (1797), when I began studying internal organs, I've seen water channels that were full, and others that were dry, revealing how little this principle was understood. Later, while treating patients and examining those who died after long illness, I noticed some drank much water, some very little, and some none at all, yet water was still found in the abdomen after death. Comparing these cases with past observations, I approached an understanding of how water exits the channels, but remained cautious about drawing definitive conclusions.

Eventually, I studied livestock for comparison: when animals were slaughtered shortly after feeding, the Net Fat was full of fluid; when they had not eaten for three or four days before slaughter, the Net Fat was dry. This confirmed beyond doubt that the Water Channels are indeed responsible for discharging fluid.

As mentioned earlier, after food enters the stomach, the solid contents remain while the essence and fluid exit via the Fluid Gate. The opening of the Fluid Gate is about the size of a chopstick. If such fine fluids can pass through it, then isn't it also possible for thin porridge to flow out?

Although the opening of the Fluid Gate is about the size of a chopstick, the stomach wall in that area is thick, and the surrounding tissues compress and narrow the passage. As a result, water and fluids can pass through, but solid food cannot.

Moreover, just to the left of the Fluid Gate, about one *fen* (a tenth of an inch) away, there is a small lump, about the size of a jujube, known as the Food Shield. Its role is to block the passage of food while allowing fluids to flow out. Only after the essence and water have drained can the remaining food ferment and cook thoroughly, gradually entering the small intestine, where it begins to transform into feces.

But how does the small intestine accomplish this transformation? Surrounding the small intestine is the Qi Chamber, a structure that envelops the gut. Between the outer wall of the intestine and the inner wall of the Qi Chamber lies the reservoir of vital Qi. It is this original Qi that digests food. (Refer to the earlier section on the Qi Chamber for further details.)

Once the feces have formed, they move into the large intestine and are eventually excreted through the anus.

This section describes the full process by which essence flows from the stomach through the Fluid Gate to generate essence and blood; how water flows from the Exquisite Duct into the Water Channels and then into the bladder to become urine; and how food passes from the stomach into the small intestine, where it is steamed and transformed into feces by the Vital Qi.

On Brain

It is said that the faculties of spirit and memory reside not in the heart, but in the brain. Originally, I hesitated to make such a claim, because even if it can be said, it may not be easily accepted in practice. Yet so many illnesses arise with causes unknown to most people that I find myself compelled to speak.

Not only do classical medical texts attribute the origin of spirit to the heart, but even Confucian discussions of morality and human nature place spirit in the heart. This is because the early theorists did not understand what the heart, located in the chest, is truly for. They did not know that on both sides of the throat are two Qi vessels that travel downward, merge in front of the lung pipe, and enter the heart. From there, the vessel turns left, exits the heart's left side, passes through the lungs, and enters the spine, this is the vessel known as the General Protective Vessel.

The General Protective Vessel connects at the front with the Qi Chamber and reproductive passage, at the back with the spine, upward with the shoulders, centrally with the kidneys, and downward with the legs. It is the reservoir of original Qi and body fluids. Since Qi flows in and out through the heart, and the heart merely serves as the pathway for this movement, how then could it possibly generate spirit or store memory?

The presence of spirit and memory resides in the brain. This is because food and drink generate Qi and blood, which nourish the muscles, while the clear refined essence is transformed into marrow. This marrow ascends through the spine into the brain, where it becomes what is called brain marrow. The structure that contains it is known as the Sea of Marrow. The bone covering the top of the head is called the Heavenly Crown.

The ears are connected to the brain, and all sounds heard are transmitted there. If brain Qi is deficient, or if there is too little brain marrow, the Qi of the brain cannot connect with the Qi of the ears, resulting in deficiency-type deafness. If the pathway between the ears and the brain is obstructed, it causes excess-type deafness.

The eyes are formed from brain fluid. The optic system, like threads, grows out from the brain, transmitting all that is seen back to the brain. The white part of the eyes is formed from brain fluid descending into the eyes, this is called brain fluid entering the eyes.

The nose is also connected to the brain. Fragrant or foul smells are transmitted directly to the brain. When the brain is invaded by wind-heat, brain fluid may flow down through the nose. This turbid and foul-smelling nasal discharge is known as brain leakage.

Observe a newborn child: the brain is not yet fully developed, the fontanel remains soft, the eyes lack coordination and alertness, the ears do not hear sounds, the nose cannot perceive smells, and the tongue cannot speak. By the age of one, the brain gradually develops, the fontanel begins to close, the ears start to register sound, the eyes gain some mobility and awareness, the nose begins to detect fragrance and odor, and the tongue can utter one or two words.

By the age of three or four, the brain marrow gradually fills out, the fontanel fully closes, the ears hear clearly, the eyes move with agility and focus, the nose perceives scents, and the child can form complete sentences.

This is why young children lack memory, the brain marrow is not yet full. Likewise, the elderly lose memory because the brain marrow gradually depletes.

Li Shizhen said that the brain is the dwelling place of the original spirit (Yuan Shen). Jin Zhengxi said that all of human memory resides in the brain. Wang Ren'an observed that when people try to recall past events, they instinctively close their eyes or look upward in reflection.

At any moment when Qi is absent from the brain, not only does the spirit vanish, but life itself ends. If Qi leaves the brain for even a single instant, death occurs in that very instant.

Try observing epilepsy, commonly known as "Lamb Wind." It occurs when the vital Qi temporarily fails to rise into the brain marrow. During a seizure, it is as if the brain has died while the person remains alive. The body is still animated, Qi is present in the abdomen, causing twitching in the limbs, but the brain is lifeless, as Qi has not reached it. The ears go deaf, the eyes roll back and stare blankly toward the sky, resembling death.

Some patients cry out just before the convulsion begins. This is because the Qi has already left the brain, and the Qi in the chest becomes confused, unsure whether to exit or enter, then suddenly bursts outward in a violent exhalation.

During the seizure, you may hear a rattling sound in the chest. This happens because body fluids accumulate in the airways. With no vital Qi in the brain to govern swallowing and spitting, fluids linger in the trachea, creating that sound.

The headache and drowsiness that follow a seizure occur because, although Qi has returned to the brain, it is still insufficient. Children who convulse after prolonged illness do so due to depleted original Qi. Adults who suddenly lose consciousness from Qi collapse experience the same thing, there is no Qi in the brain, and the patient loses all awareness and sensation.

Taken together, aren't these clear signs that the spirit and consciousness truly reside in the brain?

On Qi (energy) Blood and Pulse

As for the true nature of the pulse, I speak with honesty and clarity for future generations. Those who go against their conscience and feign mystical insight, making heartless and deceitful claims, will surely invite the wrath of Heaven.

The Qi Chamber stores vital Qi, and the Blood Chamber stores blood. The General Protective Vessel distributes Qi throughout the body from the Qi Chamber, hence its name. The General Nutrient Vessel distributes blood throughout the body from the Blood Chamber, thus its name.

The General Protective Vessel is thick and robust. It runs in front of the spine, connects with the vertebrae, and branches out to the head, face, and limbs, growing alongside the tendons and bones. It serves as the body's primary network of Qi pathways. The General Nutrient Vessel is slender and delicate. It runs in front of the General Protective Vessel, connects with it, and spreads to the head, face, and limbs, growing alongside the skin and flesh. It forms the body's system of blood vessels.

Qi moves in and out of the Qi Chamber, this exchange is what we call breathing. Actions like seeing with the eyes, hearing with the ears, turning the head, moving the body, clenching the fists, or walking, all depend on the spirit (lingji) directing the movement of Qi.

Blood flows from the Blood Chamber into the General Nutrient Vessel, which irrigates the body's entire blood vessel system. It seeps out beyond the vessels to nourish and grow the muscles.

Qi vessels grow deep alongside the tendons and bones, hidden from view and difficult to observe. Blood vessels, by contrast, run closer to the flesh and skin, making them more visible and easily exposed. Qi flows through the Qi vessels, and where Qi flows, there is movement. Blood remains contained within the blood vessels, still and unmoving.

The pulsations felt when pressing on the head, face, or limbs are all generated by Qi vessels, not blood vessels. For example, in the hollows behind the brow ridges, commonly known as the temples, there is little flesh, and the skin lies close to the bone. The pulse felt there comes from Qi vessels connected to the head and face. Between the big toe and the second toe, where flesh is sparse and the skin touches bone, the pulsation on pressure arises from Qi vessels running to the feet. Similarly, just above the transverse crease of the wrist, where the skin is thin and rests against the bone, the rhythmic beating felt is from Qi vessels reaching the hands.

Qi vessels vary in size and shape, some are thick, others thin; some run straight, others curve, depending on an individual's constitution. For instance, if the muscle below the elbow and near the wrist is thick, the Qi vessels are less exposed. If the muscle in that area is thin, the Qi vessels are more exposed and closer to the surface.

When someone contracts an external illness, such as a wind invasion, the wind enters the Qi vessels, causing them to swell. When pressed, they seem to rise toward the skin's surface. If cold enters the Qi vessels, the internal fluids congeal, blocking the flow of Qi; this results in a slower pulse when pressed. If fire invades, the heat scorches upward, and the pulse becomes rapid and forceful.

In strong individuals, where pathogenic Qi is intense, Qi accumulates in excess within the vessels. When pressed, the pulse feels full, large, and powerful. In weak individuals with deficient righteous Qi, the Qi within the vessels is scant, resulting in a pulse that feels hollow, faint, and weak.

In those with chronic illnesses and fading vitality, the original Qi becomes so depleted that it can only reach the head, face, and hands. There is no Qi left to descend downward, and thus no pulsation can be felt when pressing on the feet.

When pressing on the Qi vessels at both wrists, if the pulse feels as if it's there and yet not there, or as fine as a thread of silk, or flutters faintly and irregularly beneath the fingers, or remains still but suddenly gives a single beat, these are signs that the Qi is on the verge of collapse.

This passage explains that Qi vessels naturally vary in thickness and curvature from person to person. The length of a Qi vessel is influenced by the thickness of the wrist muscles: thicker flesh results in shorter, less exposed vessels; thinner flesh reveals longer ones. The size of the pulse when pressed helps distinguish between deficiency and excess, while the speed of the pulse, rapid or slow, helps differentiate between heat and cold conditions.

As discussed earlier, the topic was clearly the pulse, yet I refrained from naming it directly. This is because earlier scholars did not understand that the human body contains structures such as the left and right Qi Gates, the Blood Chamber, the Qi Chamber, the General Protective Vessel, the General Nutrient Vessel, the Fluid Gate, Fluid Duct, General Lifter, Food Shield, Exquisite Duct, and Water Channels. They did not know what these structures actually are in the abdomen, nor what roles they serve.

In their writings on the organs, they never clearly identified what the Pericardium is. In their meridian theories, they failed to determine what the San Jiao (Triple Burner) truly refers to, and did not clarify whether the meridians are Qi vessels or blood vessels. In pulse theory, they begin by claiming that the pulse is the "chamber of blood" that runs through all parts of the body. They assert that the pulse consists of blood vessels, and that Qi and blood circulate through them in continuous cycles.

But if we speak of circulation, for blood to flow from one point to another, there must be a space or opening to receive it. If such a space exists, it implies blood deficiency. If no space exists, then where does the blood go? The ancients did not realize that the pulse reflects the movement of Qi vessels, not blood vessels, yet they still produced numerous formulas and verses about the pulse. Though many theories were proposed, when it came to identifying the actual anatomical structures, each person gave a different account. There was no agreement.

The ancients once used twenty-seven characters to describe pulse conditions. My reason for not explaining them in depth is not that their insights lack value, but rather out of concern that future generations may no longer reply on pulse in clinical diagnosis and treatment. While it is relatively easy to use the pulse to determine life or death, it is far more difficult to identify the specific nature of a disease.

The true key to effective treatment lies in understanding Qi and blood. Whether the illness arises from external invasion or internal injury, the first step is to determine what part of the patient has been affected. It is not the internal organs, nor the muscles and bones, nor the skin and flesh that are first harmed. What is initially compromised is the Qi and blood.

Qi can be either excessive or deficient. Excess Qi refers to an overabundance of pathogenic Qi, while deficiency indicates a weakness of the righteous (vital) Qi. For patterns of righteous Qi deficiency, refer to the forty types described in the chapter on Hemiplegia, and the twenty types listed in the chapter on Pediatric Convulsions.

Blood may also be either deficient or stagnant. Blood deficiency always has an underlying cause, such as vomiting blood, nosebleeds, blood in the urine or stool, excessive bleeding from injury, heavy menstruation, uterine flooding, or postpartum hemorrhage. In cases of blood stasis, the associated symptoms can be identified through examination. Fifty such patterns are recorded later in this book for reference.

Among all conditions, blood stasis in the Blood Chamber, when stagnant blood becomes obstructed and inactive, is the most difficult to distinguish. A key sign is a fever that begins in the afternoon, worsens in the first half of the night, eases in the latter half, and is absent in the morning. This pattern indicates blood stasis in the Blood Chamber.

In milder cases, the pattern may not span all four time segments. Some may only develop a low-grade fever for about two hours around sunset. In even lighter cases, the fever may last for just a single hour. This type of fever is accompanied by a genuine sensation of body heat.

By contrast, if the body feels cool in the afternoon but experiences a brief episode of fever, it reflects a Qi deficiency pattern, typically treated with Ginseng (Ren Shen) and Astragalus (Huang Qi). If the fever occurs briefly before dawn, without any sensation of heat in the body, it suggests a pattern suitable for treatment with Ginseng (Ren Shen) and Aconite (Fu Zi).

These distinctions must not be confused or handled vaguely.

Volume I

On No Blood in the Heart

My friend Xue Wenhuang, also known as Langzhai, was a native of Tongzhou and well-versed in medicine. In the second month of the tenth year of the Daoguang reign (1830), he came to my home to bid farewell before departing for Shandong.

During our casual conversation, we touched on ancient theories regarding the origin of blood. Some claimed that the heart produces blood and the spleen governs it; others insisted that the spleen produces blood and the heart governs it. He asked which view was correct.

I replied, "Neither is accurate. Blood is formed when essence fluid enters the Blood Chamber and transforms. The heart serves as the passageway for the inflow and outflow of Qi, it contains no blood."

Langzhai responded, "Brother, what you're saying doesn't seem right. Every animal's heart contains blood, why would only the human heart be an exception?"

I asked, "Young brother, what kind of 'heart' are you referring to that has blood?"

He said, "There's a traditional formula called *Sui Xin Dan* for treating mania, which is made by mixing powdered *Gan Sui* (Euphorbia root) with pig heart blood. Doesn't that prove the pig's heart contains blood?"

I replied, "That's a misunderstanding passed down from the ancients. The blood found in the heart after it's pierced by a knife isn't originally from the heart, it's blood from the

39

thoracic cavity that flows into the heart after the injury. If you examine an unpierced heart, you'll see that there's no blood inside. I've seen this many times myself.

Look at how sheep are slaughtered. When the neck is cut without touching the heart, the heart remains free of blood. Langzhai asked, 'Then why does death come so quickly if the heart isn't pierced?'

I explained, 'It's because the thoracic cavity is full of blood. When the neck is cut, blood flows out rapidly at first. Then, the blood from the rest of the body recedes back into the chest, so the later flow is slower. Once all the blood has drained and the Qi has dispersed, death follows swiftly.

This is just like someone injured in a fight who loses too much blood. As Qi disperses and blood is lost, the person begins to convulse. The ancients called this condition *Po Shang Feng* (wound tetanus). They treated it with "wind-dispersing" formulas, often killing the patient. And since the attacker was held accountable, one death led to another, two lives lost for one mistake.

But if you understand that the true cause of death is Qi collapse due to massive blood loss, you could instead revive the Qi with strong tonics, such as half a jin of Huang Qi (Astragalus root) and four liang of Dang Shen (Codonopsis root). By saving the patient, aren't you in effect saving two lives?'

Langzhai nodded in agreement and took his leave."

Preface to Formulas

I do not discuss the concept of the Triple Burner (San Jiao), because in truth, it does not exist. The human body is divided externally into the head, face, limbs, and the network of blood vessels throughout the body. Internally, it is divided by the diaphragm into upper and lower sections. Above the diaphragm are the heart, lungs, throat, and the left and right Qi Gates; everything else lies below.

I formulated *Tong Qiao Huo Xue Tang* (Orifice-Opening and Blood-Invigorating Decoction) to treat blood stasis in the head, face, limbs, and peripheral vessels of the body. I created *Xue Fu Zhu Yu Tang* (Stasis-Expelling Decoction of the Blood Chamber) to address blood stasis in the chest, specifically, in the Blood Chamber. And I developed *Ge Xia Zhu Yu Tang* (Stasis-Expelling Decoction Below the Diaphragm) for stasis in the abdomen.

There are tens of thousands of diseases in this world. My writings are not meant to be taken as a complete medical encyclopedia. For proper pattern differentiation and diagnosis, refer to *Standards for Syndrome Identification and Treatment (Zheng Zhi Zhun Sheng)* by Wang Kentang. For prescriptions and formulas, consult *Formulas for Universal Relief (Pu Ji Fang)*, compiled under Emperor Zhu Su of the Zhou Ding. For knowledge of herbal materia medica, there is *Compendium of Materia Medica (Ben Cao Gang Mu)* by Li Shizhen. These three classics can rightfully be called foundational sources of Chinese medicine.

For those seeking something more accessible and easier to memorize, we now have the imperial edition of *Golden Mirror of Medicine (Yi Zong Jin Jian)*. For solid theoretical grounding and effective formulas, there is *On Epidemic Diseases (Wen Yi Lun)* by Wu Youke. Many other great physicians, though they had no direct view of the internal organs, still developed powerful and effective formulas for both attacking pathogens and restoring health.

I would not dare claim to have written a great medical text. But after publishing *Medical Forest Error Corrections – Visceral Illustrations*, I simply recorded several cases of Qi deficiency and blood stasis that I personally treated, so as to offer a few guiding principles for future generations. This book is not a comprehensive medical treatise. If those with little scholarly training mistakenly take it as one, it is not because I have misled them; it is because they have misunderstood me.

Diseases Treated by Tong Qiao Huo Xue Tang

Diseases Treated by Tong Qiao Huo Xue Tang (Orifice-opening and Blood-circulating Decoction)

The conditions are listed below.

Hair Loss and Alopecia

In cases of hair loss following cold-induced illness or febrile disease, most medical texts attribute the cause to blood deficiency. However, they fail to recognize that the true reason is blood stasis lodged between the skin and muscle layers, which blocks healthy blood circulation. As a result, fresh blood cannot nourish the hair, leading to hair loss. Even in cases of alopecia without prior illness, the underlying cause is still blood stasis. After taking this formula for three doses, hair loss will cease; with ten doses, new hair is certain to grow.

Eye Pain with Red Sclera

Eye pain accompanied by redness of the sclera, commonly known as "Acute Fire Eye", results from internal fire scorching the blood, causing it to accumulate in the eye. This makes the normally white sclera appear red. Whether or not cloudiness or floaters are present, begin with one dose of this formula, followed by *Jia Wei Zhi Tong Mo Yao San* (Augmented Myrrh Pain Relief Powder), taken twice daily.

The condition typically resolves completely within two to three days.

Rosacea

Red discoloration of the nose indicates blood stasis. Regardless of whether the condition has persisted for twenty or thirty years, this formula produces visible results after just three doses. With continued use, twenty to thirty doses, the condition can be fully resolved. Aside from this formula, there is no other remedy proven to be effective.

Long-standing Deafness

A small channel inside the ear connects directly to the brain. When blood stasis forms outside this channel, it creates pressure and blockage, leading to deafness. Take this formula in the evening and Tong Qi San (Qi-Regulating Powder) in the morning, two doses per day. Even deafness that has lasted twenty or thirty years may be fully restored.

Vitiligo

When blood stasis accumulates within the dermal layer of the skin, it leads to vitiligo. Taking this formula for three to five doses can halt its spread. Continued use for thirty additional doses can lead to complete healing

Purpura

When blood stasis occurs within the superficial layer of the skin, the treatment follows the same method as for vitiligo. Results are consistently swift and effective.

Purple Marks on the Face

When the face appears bruised, with blotches of dark purple or an overall purplish tone, it is caused by blood stasis. If the condition has lasted three to five years, ten doses of the formula can bring recovery. For cases lasting over a decade, twenty to thirty doses will surely cure it.

Blue or Ink-dark Marks on the Face

This is a condition caused by blood stasis, most commonly appearing on the forehead. Thirty doses of this formula can cure it. Since ancient times, there have been no effective treatments for vitiligo, purpura, purple marks, or blue-black facial discoloration, simply because the root causes were not understood.

Gingival Decay

The teeth are the extension of bone, and what nourishes them is blood. Cold Damage, epidemic diseases, pox, and internal lumps can all burn the blood. When blood becomes stagnant, the gums turn purple; when the blood dies, the gums turn black. If the blood has perished and the teeth fall out, how can the person survive? Administering cold herbs to "cool the blood" and stop bleeding only hastens death.

In such cases, give one dose of this formula in the evening, and one dose of *Xue Fu Zhu Yu Tang* (Drive Out Stasis from the Chest Decoction) in the morning. During the day, decoct 30 grams of *Huang Qi* (Astragalus Root) and sip it slowly until finished. With these three components taken daily, results can be seen in three days, marked improvement in ten, and full recovery in one month. Even if five to seven teeth have fallen out, as long as the cheeks are not ulcerated or perforated, the patient can survive.

Bad Breath (Chronic Halitosis)

When there is blood stasis in the Blood Chamber, there will inevitably be stagnation in the blood vessels. Since the airways and blood vessels are connected, how could the breath not smell foul? This is akin to the idea that wind passing through flowers carries fragrance, what lies within determines what comes out.

Take this formula in the evening, and *Xue Fu Zhu Yu Tang* (Drive Out Stasis from the Chest Decoction) in the morning. Results will appear within three to five days. Regardless of the underlying disease, if a foul odor is detected on the breath, treat it using this method.

Women's Consumptive Disorder

When a woman stops menstruating for three to four months, or even five to six months, accompanied by coughing, labored breathing, poor appetite, limb weakness, and low-grade fever that worsens in the evening, it indicates a condition of blood depletion and overexertion.

Take this prescription for three to six doses, or up to nine for severe cases. There has not been a single instance where this method failed to bring recovery.

Men's Consumptive Disorder

In the early stages of this illness, the limbs feel sore and weak. Over time, the muscles begin to waste away, appetite declines, the complexion turns pale yellow or whitish, and the patient experiences coughing with frothy sputum, irritability, afternoon tidal fevers, and heavy sweating around dawn.

Physicians are often called in to treat the condition. They typically begin by nourishing Yin, then move on to tonifying Yang. When these methods fail, they claim the body is too weak to respond to treatment and declare the case hopeless. But this thinking is laughable, such physicians fail to distinguish whether the illness arose from pre-existing weakness, or whether the weakness resulted from prolonged illness.

If the patient became sick after a serious illness such as Cold Damage or epidemic disease, and Qi and Blood were already depleted, then the disease arose from deficiency. In that case, strengthening the body will lead to recovery. But if the body was not weak at the onset and only became depleted over time, then the illness must be addressed first, once the illness resolves, vitality will naturally return.

Upon examination, if there are no exterior signs of external invasion nor interior signs of organ injury, and the symptoms are consistent with blood stasis, this is the true root. I have treated many such cases. For mild cases, nine doses of this formula are sufficient for full recovery. For more severe or longstanding cases, eighteen doses may be needed.

If, after three doses, the patient still presents with Qi deficiency, decoct 24 grams (eight qian) of Huang Qi (Astragali Radix / Astragalus Root) daily and sip the decoction slowly throughout the day. This approach combines resolution and restoration. But if Qi is not significantly weak, there is no need to add Huang Qi, the vital energy will return naturally once the illness is resolved.

Illness Triggered by the Change of Solar Terms

Regardless of the specific illness, if symptoms consistently flare up at the change of a Solar Term (seasonal transition), the root cause is blood stasis. How can we be sure? Because cases of hematemesis caused by blood stasis often relapse at these seasonal junctures as well. This pattern confirms the link. With three doses of this formula, the recurrence can be stopped.

Pediatric Gan Syndrome (malnutrition)

Pediatric Gan Syndrome (malnutrition, 19 Types Identified)

In the early stage of Gan disease in children, the urine appears cloudy like rice water, and tidal fevers develop in the afternoon. Over time, blue veins become prominent, the belly swells and hardens, the complexion turns bluish-yellow, muscles waste away, the skin looks dry and withered, and the child's eyes become dull and lifeless.

In classical Chinese medicine, these symptoms were viewed as *Lao Bing* (consumptive disease) in adults and *Gan Ji* (gan accumulation) in children. As more specific presentations were observed, additional descriptors were added, based on either the affected organ or the symptomatic expression, resulting in named conditions such as Spleen Gan, Gan Diarrhea, Gan Swelling, Gan Dysentery, Liver Gan, Heart Gan, Gan Thirst, Lung Gan, Kidney Gan, Gan Heat, Brain Gan, Eye Gan, Nasal Gan, Dental Gan, Spinal Gan, Roundworm Gan, Innocent Gan, Dingxi Gan, and Emesis-Related Gan. Nineteen such variants were classified, and fifty formulas were devised to treat them.

Many of these traditional prescriptions relied heavily on extremely cold substances like Gardenia (Zhi Zi), Coptis (Huang Lian), Antelope Horn (Ling Yang Jiao), and Gypsum (Shi Gao), based on the theory that overfeeding on rich, greasy, and sweet foods caused food stagnation in the stomach. This stagnation was believed to slow digestive movement, damage the spleen and stomach, and generate internal heat over time. The resulting "accumulated heat" was thought to consume Qi and blood and scorch the body's fluids, thus requiring intensely cold herbs to cool and purge the heat.

In my earlier clinical experience, I prescribed formulas following this traditional pattern, yet saw no therapeutic effect. Upon deeper reflection, I carefully reviewed the classical theories and found contradictions. If the root cause is indeed unregulated feeding and food stagnation in the middle burner, then the pathology is stagnation, and it is inappropriate to use such harshly cold herbs. If the damage to the digestive process leads to heat, it is likely a case of deficient heat, not excessive heat, and still not suitable for strong cooling herbs.

Later, through close clinical observation, I found that many of these children developed tidal fever in the afternoon that worsened by evening, an indicator of blood stasis. The so-called "exposed sinews" were not sinews at all, but visible veins on the surface of the skin, bluish in color due to stagnant blood within. As the condition progressed, the abdomen became enlarged, firm, and lumpy, clear signs of coagulated blood and stagnant accumulation.

For such cases, I achieved reliable results using the following approach:

– *Tong Qiao Huo Xue Tang* (Orifice-Opening and Blood-Circulating Decoction) to unblock the blood vessels;

– *Xue Fu Zhu Yu Tang* (Expelling Stasis from the Blood Chamber Decoction) to clear the afternoon tidal fever;

– *Ge Xia Zhu Yu Tang* (Expelling Stasis from Below the Diaphragm Decoction) to dissolve the abdominal masses.

By rotating these three formulas appropriately, I have never failed to produce therapeutic effects.

Tong Qiao Huo Xue Tang

Tong Qiao Huo Xue Tang (Orifice-opening and Blood-circulating Decoction)

Ingredients:

Pin Yin	Latin Name	English Name	Amount (grams)
Chi Shao	Paeoniae Radix Rubra	Red Peony Root	3
Chuan Xiong	Chuanxiong Rhizoma	Cnidium	3
Tao Ren	Persicae Semen (mashed)	Peach Kernel (mashed)	9
Hong Hua	Carthemi Flos	Safflower	9
Lao Cong	Allium fistulosum	Green Onion	3 whole
Sheng Jiang	Zingiberis Rhizoma Recens	Fresh Ginger	9
Da Zao	Jujubae Fructus	Jujube (Date)	7 pieces

Pin Yin	Latin Name	English Name	Amount (grams)
Huang Jiu	Rice Wine	Yellow Wine	250
She Xiang	Moschus	Musk	0.15

Preparation

Boil the seven herbs above with 500 grams of yellow rice wine until the liquid is reduced to one cup. Strain out the herb residue, then add She Xiang (Moschus / Musk) directly into the decoction. Bring the mixture to a boil two more times. Take the medicine warm, just before bedtime.

Note that the volume of yellow wine may vary slightly depending on the region or manufacturer. It is better to use slightly more, an extra 100g, than to use too little. Once boiled down to one cup, the alcohol content is greatly reduced and the wine loses its characteristic smell, making it tolerable even for those who usually cannot consume alcohol.

Be especially cautious with She Xiang (Moschus / Musk), as it is often adulterated. One 3 grams of authentic musk is frequently mixed with up to 60 grams of counterfeit product, and it is difficult for most people to tell the difference. Since She Xiang is the most critical component of this formula, it is worth the additional cost to obtain a high-quality, authentic product. Ideally, try to purchase what is known as *Dang Men*

Zi, musk taken directly from the opening of the gland, which is considered the most potent.

Dosage Guidelines

- Adults: Take one dose each night for three consecutive nights. After skipping one night, repeat with another three consecutive doses.
- Children aged 7–8: Take one dose every other night.
- Children aged 2–3: Take one dose every three nights.

Note: The same portion of She Xiang can be decocted and reused for up to three doses before replacing it with a new one.

Formula Rhyme

To open the orifices, fine musk leads the way;

Peach kernel, safflower, jujube, scallion, and ginger stay.

Chuan Xiong with wine, Chi Shao in blend,

The top prescription to unblock meridians end to end.

Jia Wei Zhi Tong Mo Yao San

Jia Wei Zhi Tong Mo Yao San (Myrrha Painkiller Plus)

Used to treat early-stage eye pain and redness of the sclera, which later develops into cloudiness or visual obstructions.

Ingredients

Pin Yin	Latin Name	English Name	Amount (grams)
Mo Yao	Myrrha	Myrrh	9
Xue Jie	Calamus Draco	Dragon Blood	9
Da Huang	Rhei Radix Et Rhizoma	Rhubarb Root	6
Mang Xiao	Natrii Sulfas	Mirabilite	6
Shi Jue Ming	Haliotidis Concha	Abalone Shell	9

Preparation and Usage: Grind all ingredients into fine powder, mix thoroughly, and divide into four equal doses. Take one dose with clear tea, morning and evening. This has been the sole enduring formula for external eye conditions for thousands of years.

Tong Qi San (Qi Moving Powder)

Formulated to treat deafness so severe that even thunder cannot be heard. I created this prescription when I was thirty years old.

Ingredients

Pin Yin	Latin Name	English Name	Amount (grams)
Chai Hu	Bupleuri Radix	Hare's Ear Root	30
Xiang Fu	Cyperi Rhizoma	Cyperus	30
Chuan Xiong	Chuanxiong Rhizoma	Cnidium	15

Preparation and Usage: Grind all ingredients into a fine powder, mix evenly, and take 9 grams with warm water, morning and night.

Diseases Treated by Xue Fu Zhu Yu Tang

Diseases Treated by Xue Fu Zhu Yu Tang (Expelling Stasis from the Blood Chamber Decoction)

The conditions are listed below.

Headache

If a headache is caused by an external contraction, it will always present with symptoms like fever and aversion to cold, releasing the exterior resolves it.

If it is due to internal heat accumulation, there will be signs such as a dry tongue and thirst, Cheng Qi Decoctions can bring relief.

If it stems from Qi deficiency, the pain will feel dull or indistinct, tonifying Qi with Ginseng (Ren Shen) and Astragalus (Huang Qi) will be effective.

But if a patient presents with none of these, no exterior symptoms, no interior excess, no signs of Qi deficiency or phlegm-fluid retention, and the headache comes and goes unpredictably while hundreds of formulas fail, then one dose of this specific formula will bring a cure.

Chest Pain

Chest pain located in the front of the chest can be resolved with *Mu Jin San* (Saussurea and Curcuma Powder). If the pain radiates to the back, *Gua Lou Xie Bai Bai Jiu Tang* (Trichosanthes Fruit, Chinese Chive, and Aged Rice Wine Decoction) is effective. When chest pain arises from Cold Damage (Shang Han), formulas containing *Gua Lou* (Trichosanthis Fructus), *Xian Xiong Tang* (Chest Obstruction Decoction), or *Chai Hu* (Bupleuri Radix) can bring relief. In cases of sudden, acute chest pain where the above formulas prove ineffective, administering a single dose of this specific prescription will stop the pain immediately.

Chest Cannot Tolerate Any Pressure

Mr. Lin, Governor of Jiangxi Province, age 74, had been ill for seven years. He could only fall asleep at night with his chest fully exposed; even the light pressure of a single layer of cloth over his chest would prevent sleep. I was summoned to treat him, and after five doses of this formula, he was completely cured.

Chest Requires Pressure to Sleep

A 22-year-old woman had suffered from this condition for two years: she could only fall asleep at night if her maid sat on her chest to apply pressure. I prescribed the same formula used in the previous case, and she was cured after three doses.

If asked about the causes of illness in both of these cases, how should one respond?

Sweating at Dawn

Sweating after waking is known as *spontaneous sweating*. Waking due to sweating is referred to as *night sweating*, which drains a person's Qi and blood. This distinction has held true for a thousand years. Yet there are cases where treatments aimed at tonifying Qi, securing the exterior, nourishing Yin, or clearing internal heat not only fail to help but actually worsen the condition. This is because the role of *blood stasis* in causing both spontaneous and night sweating is often overlooked. In such cases, just one or two doses of *Xue Fu Zhu Yu Tang* (Drive Out Blood Stasis in the Mansion of Blood Decoction) can stop the sweating.

Food Travels Down the Right Side of the Chest

Normally, food descends through the esophagus along the center of the chest. However, in some individuals, after entering the pharynx, food appears to travel down the right side of the chest. The esophagus lies behind the trachea but curves forward below the lungs, passes in front of them, and then exits the thoracic cavity by passing through the diaphragm into the abdomen. The trachea remains centered, but when there is blood stasis in the *Blood Chamber* (Xue Fu), the esophagus may be displaced to the right.

When the condition is mild, it is easier to treat, as eating remains largely unaffected. In more severe cases, the esophagus becomes compressed, bent, and narrowed, making food passage difficult. This formula can bring relief, but a complete cure is often hard to achieve.

Internal Heat with Cold Exterior (Lantern Disease)

When the body feels cold on the outside but burns with heat inside, it is referred to as *Lantern Disease*. This pattern is rooted in internal blood stasis.

If mistaken for deficient heat, the more one tonifies, the more stagnation builds. If mistaken for excess heat, the more one tries to clear fire, the more coagulation results.

With just two to three doses of this formula, blood circulation becomes smooth and the internal heat naturally subsides.

Depressive Stifling

When even trivial matters weigh heavily on the mind and one cannot feel at ease, it is often due to blood stasis. This condition can be resolved with three doses of the prescribed formula.

Irritability During Illness

A person who is usually calm and even-tempered but becomes irritable when ill is likely experiencing blood stasis. One to two doses of the prescribed formula will certainly resolve the condition.

Excessive Dreaming at Night

Experiencing many dreams during sleep is often caused by blood stasis. One to two doses of this formula can fully resolve the condition, there is no better alternative treatment.

Hiccups

Hiccups arise when blood stasis in the *Blood Chamber* compresses the airway that forms above the heart, where the left and right *Qi passages* converge into a single tracheal channel. This obstruction prevents inhaled air from descending and instead forces it upward, resulting in hiccups.

In severe cases, when the trachea becomes fully blocked by stasis and air cannot enter or exit, the patient may suffocate and die.

Ancient physicians, unaware of the true cause, attempted treatments with formulas such as *Ju Pi Zhu Ru Tang* (Tangerine Peel and Bamboo Shavings Decoction), *Cheng Qi Tang* (Order the Qi Decoction), *Du Qi Tang* (Governor Qi Decoction), *Ding Xiang Shi Di Tang* (Clove and Persimmon Calyx Decoction), *Fu Zi Li Zhong Tang* (Aconite to Regulate the Middle Decoction), *Sheng Jiang Xie Xin Tang* (Fresh Ginger Drain the Epigastrium Decoction), *Xuan Fu Dai Zhe Tang* (Inula and Hematite Decoction), as well as *Da Xian Xiong Tang* and *Xiao Xian Xiong Tang* (Major and Minor Chest Congestion Decoctions), but none proved effective.

It was even believed that hiccups arising from Cold Damage or Epidemic Disease were always fatal. Due to the lack of effective treatments, physicians in the past often abandoned such cases.

No matter the origin, Cold Damage, epidemic illness, or other miscellaneous diseases, when hiccups appear, administer this formula immediately. Whether the condition is mild or severe, just one dose will produce clear results. This is a method I have personally validated through clinical experience.

Choking When Drinking Water

Choking immediately upon drinking water is caused by blood stagnation in the epiglottis. This formula is extremely effective for such cases.

The explanations given by earlier physicians were all mistaken, I provide a detailed clarification in the section on Pox Disorders.

Insomnia

When one cannot fall asleep at night, and conventional treatments with formulas that calm the spirit and nourish the blood prove ineffective, this prescription yields remarkable results.

Infant Night Crying

Why does the child cry only at night but not during the day? The cause is blood stasis. One to two doses of this formula will bring complete recovery.

Palpitations and Rapid Heartbeat

For cases of palpitations and tachycardia where formulas such as *Gui Pi Tang* (Restore the Spleen Decoction) or other spirit-calming prescriptions fail to produce results, this formula is unfailingly effective, like hitting the target with every shot.

Restlessness at Night

The patient feels restless through the night, lying down only to sit up again, then sitting up only to feel the urge to lie back down. The night passes without a moment of peace. In severe cases, the person may toss and roll continuously in bed.

This condition is caused by blood stasis in the *Blood Chamber*. Taking ten or more doses of this formula can fully eliminate the root of the disorder.

Anger or Sulking

Unprovoked or frequent anger, or silent brooding without an obvious cause, is often the result of blood stasis in the Blood Chamber. It should not be treated with Qi-regulating formulas. This prescription, however, brings rapid and reliable results.

Retching

When retching occurs without any accompanying symptoms, it is often caused by blood stasis. Using this formula to invigorate the blood can stop the retching immediately.

Nighttime Fever Episodes

Each night, the body experiences a wave of internal heat accompanied by warmth of the skin, lasting for a short period. A single dose of this formula is sufficient to resolve the condition; in more severe cases, two doses will bring complete relief.

Xue Fu Zhu Yu Tang

Xue Fu Zhu Yu Tang (Expelling Stasis from Blood Chamber Decoction)

Ingredients

Pin Yin	Latin Name	English Name	Amount (grams)
Dang Gui	Angelicae Sinensis Radix	Chinese Angelica Root	9
Sheng Di Huang	Rehmanniae Radix	Rehmanniae Root	9

Pin Yin	Latin Name	English Name	Amount (grams)
Tao Ren	Persicae Semen (mashed)	Peach Kernel (mashed)	12
Hong Hua	Carthemi Flos	Safflower	9
Zhi Ke	Aurantii Fructus	Bitter Orange	6
Chi Shao	Paeoniae Radix Rubra	Red Peony Root	6
Chai Hu	Bupleuri Radix	Hare's Ear Root	3
Gan Cao	Glycyrrhizae Radix	Licorice Root	6
Jie Geng	Platycodi Radix	Balloon Flower Root	4.5
Chuan Xiong	Chuanxiong Rhizoma	Cnidium	4.5
Niu Xi	Cyathulae Radix	Cyathula Root	9

Preparation: Boil them with water and drink the decoction 3 times a day.

Formula Rhyme

Dang Gui, Sheng Di, Tao Ren too,

Hong Hua, Zhi Qiao, Chi Shao through.

Chai Hu, Gan Cao, Jie Geng stay,

Chuan Xiong, Niu Xi guide the way.

To move the blood and ease its flow,

Downward it goes, no strain, no woe.

Diseases Treated by Ge Xia Zhu Yu Tang

Diseases Treated by Ge Xia Zhu Yu Tang (Expelling Stasis from Under the Diaphragm Decoction)

The conditions are listed below.

Mass Formation

When it comes to the condition of mass formation, there is no need to revisit the ancient classifications such as the Five Accumulations, Six Gatherings, Seven Masses, or Eight Tumors, nor to spend time refuting those old theories, it would be unnecessarily tedious. Instead, let us ask a simple question: what can form a mass in the abdomen?

If the mass is located in the stomach, it must be food. If in the intestines, it is likely hardened stool. However, when a mass persists for a long time and the patient's diet remains unchanged, it is clear that the mass is not within the stomach or intestines, but outside of them.

Outside the gastrointestinal tract, there is nothing but Qi and blood. Qi travels through its own channels, and blood flows through blood vessels. Qi is formless and cannot congeal into a mass. Therefore, anything that forms a tangible mass must be blood.

Blood exposed to cold will congeal into a lump. Blood exposed to heat will become thickened and scorched into a mass. If congealing occurs in vertical vessels, the mass will form in a vertical strip; if in horizontal vessels, a horizontal strip. When both vertical and horizontal vessels are affected, the coagulated blood will connect into a sheet. Over time, this sheet thickens and hardens into a solid mass.

Since It Is a Blood Mass, There Should Be Fever. Whenever there is blood stasis in the *Blood Chamber* (Xue Fu), fever must be present. This is because the Blood Chamber is the root of all blood in the body, and stagnation there can be fatal. In contrast, when blood stasis occurs in the abdomen, fever is usually absent. The abdomen is considered the end branch of the blood network, while stasis there can lead to accumulation, it does not endanger life.

Regardless of where the mass is located, whether under the left or right ribs, to the left or right of the navel, above or below the navel, or whether it presents as a pulsating mass when pressed, this formula can be used effectively. Results are often seen quickly and reliably.

Patients with mild conditions need fewer doses; those with more severe cases require more. In all cases, discontinue the medicine once the condition resolves, do not continue taking it unnecessarily.

If the patient has deficient Qi and is too weak to withstand the dispersing and reducing action of the formula, simply add 9 to 15 grams of *Dang Shen* (Codonopsis Radix). There's no need to adhere rigidly to exact proportions in such adjustments.

Pediatric Abdominal Masses

In children, abdominal lumps accompanied by a distended belly and prominent bluish veins are almost always caused by blood stasis. To treat this, alternate among three formulas: this one, *Tong Qiao Huo Xue Tang*, and *Xue Fu Zhu Yu Tang*. When taken in rotation over the course of a month or so, treatment is consistently successful.

Fixed-Point Abdominal Pain

When abdominal pain is confined to a constant, unchanging spot, the underlying cause is usually blood stasis. This formula is exceptionally effective for resolving such pain.

Abdominal Heaviness That Shifts During Sleep

At night the patient feels a heavy mass inside the abdomen: when lying on the left side it sinks to the left, and when lying on the right side it sinks to the right. This presentation indicates blood stasis within the abdomen. Use this formula as the principal treatment, adding other herbs as needed to address any accompanying patterns.

Early-Morning Diarrhea (Kidney Diarrhea)

Patients who pass loose stools two or three times just before dawn have long been diagnosed with "Kidney Diarrhea" and treated as if the root were kidney deficiency, commonly with *Er Shen Wan* ("Two Immortals Pill") or *Si Shen Wan* ("Four Immortals Pill"). These remedies often fail, leaving the condition unresolved for years.

The true culprit is usually overlooked: blood stasis along the pancreas. When the patient lies down, this congealed blood blocks the Fluid Gate (*Jin Men*), preventing fluids from draining as they should. Instead, the water diverts through the pylorus into the small intestine, where it mixes with waste and produces watery stools, hence the repeated bowel movements in the early morning hours.

By using this formula to disperse the pancreatic blood stasis, the Fluid Gate reopens, normal fluid passage is restored, and the diarrhea stops. Most cases resolve completely after three to five doses.

Chronic Diarrhea

Chronic Diarrhea for a long time without effective treatment using any other formulas is because of too much blood stasis on the General Lifter (Pancreas). Also use this formula to treat it.

Ge Xia Zhu Yu Tang

Ge Xia Zhu Yu Tang (Expelling Stasis from Under the Diaphragm Decoction)

Pin Yin	Latin Name	English Name	Amount (grams)
Wu Ling Zhi	Faeces Trogopterori	Pteropus, Trogopterus	6
Dang Gui	Angelicae Sinensis Radix	Chinese Angelica Root	9

Medical Forest Error Corrections

Pin Yin	Latin Name	English Name	Amount (grams)
Chuan Xiong	Chuanxiong Rhizoma	Cnidium	6
Tao Ren	Persicae Semen (mashed)	Peach Kernel (mashed)	9
Dan Pi	Moutan Cortex	Tree Peony Bark	6
Chi Shao	Paeoniae Radix Rubra	Red Peony Root	6
Wu Yao	Linderae Radix	Lindera Root	6
Yan Hu Suo (Yuan Hu)	Rhizoma Corydalis	Corydalis	3
Gan Cao	Glycyrrhizae Radix	Licorice Root	9
Xiang Fu	Cyperi Rhizoma	Cyperus	4.5
Hong Hua	Carthemi Flos	Safflower	9
Zhi Ke	Aurantii Fructus	Bitter Orange	4.5

Preparation and Usage:

Boil them together with water and drink the decoction

70

Formula Rhyme

Tao Ren, Mu Dan clear the way,

Chi Shao, Wu Yao, Yuan Hu stay.

Dang Gui, Chuan Xiong, Ling Zhi blend,

Hong Hua, Zhi Qiao, their powers send.

Xiang Fu soothes what's stuck inside,

Blood flows with peace, no pain to hide.

Volume 2

Preface to On Hemiplegia

When medical scholars compose theoretical works, their highest aim should be a sincere wish to relieve suffering and benefit the world. To fulfill this mission, one must personally treat the illness in question and repeatedly verify the methods, ensuring they are unfailingly effective, before passing them down to future generations. If any aspect of a condition remains unclear, it is better to leave it for future physicians to clarify, rather than force conclusions.

It is absolutely unacceptable to invent theories or create formulas based on speculation alone, driven by ambition or reputation, without grounding them in clinical experience. If one fails to understand the root of a disease, and the prescriptions do not match the condition, then even with the intention to save lives, one may tragically cause harm. How can one not feel fear in the face of such responsibility?

In fields like Cold Damage, Epidemic Disorders, Miscellaneous Diseases, and Gynecology, our predecessors each had their strengths. Their formulas often matched the conditions and yielded swift, effective results. Occasional errors were like minor flaws in flawless jade, regrettable, but not destructive.

But hemiplegia stands apart. Of the more than four hundred medical authors who came before me, only a handful attempted to build theories around this condition, and among them, not one clearly identified its root cause. How can one develop a correct treatment if the origin of the illness is misunderstood? Mistakes are inevitable.

In my youth, I encountered this illness and first followed the teachings of the *Ling Shu*, *Su Wen*, and Zhang Zhongjing. But the treatments failed. Then I turned to the methods of Liu Hejian, Li Dongyuan, and Zhu Danxi, yet still found no success. After many attempts and much frustration, I nearly despaired.

I reflected deeply: Zhang Zhongjing wrote *Treatise on Cold Damage*, and Wu Youke composed *Treatise on Epidemic Diseases*, each an original work drawn from personal insight, without merely quoting classical texts. I too held a heartfelt desire to save lives, but lacked the ability to truly serve the world.

Whenever I encountered this illness, I studied it with great care, examining whether the Qi and Blood were flourishing or depleted, and discerning whether the meridians were open or obstructed. Over the course of forty years, this diligent inquiry has yielded significant insight.

I have long wished to share these findings publicly, to offer help to future generations. Yet I hesitated, fearful of overstepping, of using my limited understanding to challenge the theories of past masters, or to establish new treatments and invite reproach.

But a friend once told me: "You have a sincere heart and genuine insight. You have repeatedly tested this formula with consistent success. What you offer fills in the gaps left by our predecessors and relieves the suffering of those to come. In doing so, you not only serve future generations but also bring honor to those who came before. What fault is there in that?"

Encouraged by his words, I cast aside my shame over any lack of scholarly brilliance. I have recorded, in detail, the cases of hemiplegia, leg paralysis and atrophy, convulsions, and muscle spasms in men, women, and children. I describe the causes of these disorders, their clinical manifestations, the repeatedly verified treatments, and the varying degrees of difficulty in managing them.

I have also identified and clarified errors in the traditional interpretations of pulse patterns, internal organs, and meridian theory. Where necessary, I have illustrated these findings with diagrams and clearly explained the progression of symptoms before and after treatment, leaving room for more enlightened minds to expand upon this work in the future.

Is this not, in its own way, a modest contribution to the advancement of medical knowledge?

Medical Forest Error Corrections

On Hemiplegia

Hemiplegia is fundamentally one and the same condition, yet the theories proposed by various medical authorities differ significantly.

The earliest account appears in the *Ling Shu Jing* (*The Spiritual Pivot*), which states that due to Qi deficiency, external pathogenic Qi lodges in one side of the body. As it penetrates deeper, it invades the internal realms of Qi and Blood. Once the body's Qi and Blood are weakened, the Righteous Qi disperses, leaving only the pathogenic Qi behind, resulting in partial withering of the body. This "partial withering" is what we now call hemiplegia.

The *Su Wen* (*Basic Questions*) explains that external Wind invades the shu-points of the internal organs. This form of Wind invasion results in what is known as "Wind Stroke with one-sided paralysis." Zhang Zhongjing also stated that illnesses caused by Wind should lead to hemiplegia. These three classical texts all share a common theme: Wind is the primary cause of the condition.

Later, Liu Hejian observed that the classical theories and formulas had limited clinical success, so he proposed a new perspective. In his view, stroke does not result from internal Wind arising from Liver Wood, nor from external Wind invasion. Rather, it stems from an imbalanced lifestyle, irregular work and rest, that leads to excessive internal Fire. When internal fluids are depleted, they can no longer restrain the Fire. The result is loss of clarity in the mind, sudden collapse, and unconsciousness. His theory emphasizes internal Fire as the root cause.

76

Li Dongyuan, seeing contradictions between Liu Hejian's theory and his formulas, established yet another view. He argued that stroke arises from Qi deficiency, which allows external Wind to invade the body. This condition tends to occur after the age of forty, rarely affecting the strong and vigorous, but occasionally appearing in overweight individuals with deficient Qi. His system categorizes stroke into four types: Fu-organ (Yang organ) stroke, Zang-organ (Yin organ) stroke, Blood Vessel stroke, and Meridian stroke. His core thesis is that the root of the disease lies in a deficiency of internal Qi that allows external Wind to enter and cause disorder.

Zhu Danxi, observing that Li Dongyuan's prescriptions did not align with the actual disease presentations, proposed a different theory. He noted that in the cold, dry climate of the Northwest, one could encounter true Wind Stroke (*Zhong Feng*), but in the humid Southeast, such cases were not genuine Wind Stroke. He believed that the root lay in prior deficiencies of Qi and Blood, which allowed dampness to generate phlegm; phlegm then gave rise to heat, and heat in turn stirred internal Wind. His theory centered on phlegm, making dampness and phlegm the foundation of his understanding.

Wang Andao, picking up on Danxi's statement that the dampness of the Southeast did not produce true Wind Stroke, concluded that what the *Ling Shu*, *Su Wen*, and Zhang Zhongjing described were cases of true Wind Stroke, while the theories of Liu Hejian, Li Dongyuan, and Zhu Danxi pertained only to pseudo-stroke or stroke-like conditions.

Yu Tianmin, however, disagreed with Wang Andao's distinction between true and pseudo stroke. He argued that regardless of geographic region, the condition arises from a combination of Qi deficiency, dampness, phlegm, fire, and Wind, all working together. Where, he asked, is the clear boundary between true and pseudo stroke?

Only Zhang Jingyue put forth an insight that rose above the rest. He proposed that hemiplegia is generally due to Qi deficiency and even redefined the disease, shifting the term "Wind Stroke" (*Zhong Feng*) away from its association with Wind altogether. Instead, he rooted his discussion in the *Nei Jing*'s theory of *Jue Ni* (inversion syndromes), and analyzed the condition through the lenses of cold and heat, blood deficiency, and the symptomatic patterns across the twelve meridians.

Unfortunately, the symptom descriptions in his writings do not fully match clinical reality, and his formulas often failed to produce results. This was likely due to his limited firsthand experience in treating the condition.

The causes of hemiplegia, as proposed by many esteemed physicians throughout history, have revolved around Wind, Fire, Qi, and Phlegm. Accordingly, the formulas they developed aim to dispel Wind, clear Fire, regulate Qi, or resolve Phlegm.

Some have argued that hemiplegia arises from a deficiency of Qi and Blood, which allows Wind to invade. In such cases, they add Qi- and Blood-tonifying herbs to formulas that also disperse Wind and clear Fire. Others believe the root is a deficiency of Yin, again permitting Wind to invade, and thus prescribe Yin-nourishing and Kidney-tonifying herbs supported by Qi-regulating and phlegm-transforming agents.

Some lean more heavily on supplementation, others on purgation, yet all claim they are applying a balanced strategy of both attacking and replenishing, each according to their own experience. However, when these treatments are followed today, they often fail to produce results.

Rather than openly questioning the flaws in ancient theories, many modern practitioners attempt to justify the failure by saying that classical formulas no longer suit present-day illnesses, or that the vital Qi of people today differs from that of the ancients.

But if ancient formulas were truly unsuitable for modern ailments, why do formulas for Cold Damage, like *Ma Huang Tang* (Ephedra Decoction), *Cheng Qi Tang* (Order the Qi Decoction), *Xian Xiong Tang* (Chest Binding Decoction), and *Chai Hu Tang* (Bupleurum Decoction), still produce immediate and reliable results? And why do stroke formulas aimed at dispelling Wind, transforming phlegm, or using *Qin Jiao* (Gentiana Macrophylla Root) and *San Hua Tang* (Three-Transformation Decoction) so often fail?

The truth is this: the ancients developed their formulas by two distinct methods. The effective formulas came from firsthand clinical experience, repeatedly tested and refined through real cases. The ineffective ones were based on speculation, formed by discussing theories and imagining disease mechanisms rather than observing them.

How can anyone expect to truly understand the root of a disease if their reasoning is purely theoretical? Why does hemiplegia cause facial paralysis? Why slurred speech and drooling? Why dry stools with frequent urination? There has never been a clear, systematic explanation, confusion and conjecture, past and present alike.

To treat an illness that has already robbed a patient of half their vital Qi with purging and aggressive formulas, how could that not be a serious error?

At its core, the fault does not lie with the physician administering the treatment, but with the authors who constructed flawed theories and passed them down. Alas, how grave a matter this is, and yet how casually some still rely on guesswork, assumptions, and wishful thinking!

Hemiplegia Differentiation

Some have asked: "You challenge the traditional theories of Wind, Fire, Dampness, and Phlegm in the etiology of hemiplegia. Do you have any evidence to support your position?"

To answer, let us begin with Zhang Zhongjing's *Treatise on Cold Damage*, in the chapter on Wind Invasion. It states that when Wind enters the body, the patient will experience headache and body aches, fever with aversion to cold, retching, and spontaneous sweating. In the *Essential Prescriptions of the Golden Chamber*, Wind-Cold is said to cause nasal congestion, sneezing, a heavy cough, and clear nasal discharge. The chapter on Stroke in the same text also states that Wind-induced illness can lead to hemiplegia.

Now I ask: what kind of Wind, and by what mechanism, causes headache and body pain, fever and chills, retching, and sweating? What kind of Wind causes nasal blockage, sneezing, severe coughing, and runny nose? And what kind of Wind causes hemiplegia?

If hemiplegia is truly caused by Wind, then Wind must invade from the exterior, through the skin, into the meridians. In that case, there should be observable signs of disease progressing from the exterior to the interior.

But from my clinical experience treating this condition, I have found that at the onset of hemiplegia, patients do not show exterior symptoms such as fever, chills, headache, body aches, sore eyes, dry nasal passages, or alternating cold and heat. The absence of these exterior signs is clear evidence that Wind has not invaded the body.

Furthermore, the theories centered on Wind, Fire, Dampness, and Phlegm are often vague and contradictory. Whether these pathogenic factors arise externally or internally, they must affect the meridians. But the meridians contain only Qi and Blood. If Wind, Fire, Dampness, or Phlegm were obstructing Qi and Blood, there should be clear symptoms of pain.

Pain, however, is the hallmark of *Bi Syndrome*, a condition of painful obstruction, not of hemiplegia. Hemiplegia presents without pain. Over the course of my life, having treated more cases of hemiplegia than any other condition, I have never seen a case caused by *Bi Syndrome* with painful obstruction.

From this line of reasoning, we can conclude: hemiplegia is not the result of Wind, Fire, Dampness, or Phlegm invasion.

Cause of Hemiplegia

Some have asked me, "You claim that hemiplegia arises from the depletion of Yuan Qi (Original Vitality). But why does the condition only appear once 50% of it is lost? I'd like to hear your explanation."

I replied: Yuan Qi is stored within the Qi vessels and distributed throughout the body, half to the left side, half to the right. Every action we perform, standing, sitting, walking, turning, depends entirely on Yuan Qi. When Yuan Qi is abundant, the body has strength. When it is depleted, the body weakens. When it is completely lost, life ceases.

If one has ten parts of Yuan Qi and loses only two, eight remain, four for each side of the body. No illness appears. But if five parts are lost and only five remain, each half of the body receives just two and a half. At this stage, although hemiplegia has not yet developed, symptoms of Qi deficiency are already present. However, since there is neither pain nor discomfort, the patient remains unaware.

Once Yuan Qi is diminished, the meridians naturally become hollow, creating internal gaps. In such a state, it is inevitable that Qi will shift and merge toward one side. If the right side's 2.5 parts of Qi merge into the left, the right side is left without Qi. If the left side's 2.5 parts merge into the right, the left side is depleted. A body part without Qi cannot move, and immobility of one side is called hemiplegia (*ban shen bu sui*). The term "bu sui" means the body no longer follows the will.

When this Qi shift occurs during sleep, the patient is unaware, yet upon waking, they cannot turn over. If the Qi merges from one side to the other while the patient is awake, they may feel a current flowing from the affected side to the healthy one, so forceful it sounds louder than rushing water.

If the Qi shifts while seated, the body leans and collapses. If it happens while walking, one side lacks Qi and strength, leading to a fall. People often think hemiplegia was caused by the fall. But they do not realize: it was not the fall that caused the hemiplegia, it was the depletion of Yuan Qi that caused both the hemiplegia and the fall.

Facial Droop Differentiation

Facial Droop (Deviation Of The Mouth And Eyes) Differentiation

Some have asked: "If hemiplegia is not caused by Wind, then why does it result in facial deviation, where the mouth and eyes appear slanted?"

I replied: The ancient term "facial deviation" was coined because physicians of the past failed to examine the condition with sufficient clinical care. What appears to be slanting is not truly a deviation in the structural sense.

In cases of hemiplegia, the affected side of the face lacks Qi. Without Qi, the muscles on that side shrink. The eye on the affected side loses strength and cannot fully open, causing the inner corner to pull downward. The mouth on the same side loses strength and cannot open properly, while the opposite corner lifts. The upper and lower features appear misaligned. At a glance, it looks like the face is slanted, but in truth, it is not a lateral deviation.

From my clinical experience, I've observed that when the left side of the body is paralyzed, the face appears to droop toward the right; when the right side is paralyzed, the face appears to droop toward the left. This pattern is difficult for most to grasp, and unfortunately, there are no classical texts that explain it.

Why do the meridians of the left side of the body ascend to the right side of the head and face, while those from the right side ascend to the left? What is the significance of this crossover between left and right?

I do not dare offer a final conclusion. I leave it to those of greater insight to investigate this phenomenon thoroughly and contribute further understanding.

Some have asked: "Is facial deviation, where the mouth and eyes appear slanted, always caused by a lack of Yuan Qi on one side of the face?"

I replied: The explanation I gave earlier applies specifically to cases of facial deviation that occur alongside hemiplegia.

However, in otherwise strong and healthy individuals, if facial deviation appears suddenly without accompanying hemiplegia, the cause is different, it is a disorder of the meridians being obstructed by Wind. When Wind obstructs the meridians, Yuan Qi cannot rise to the head and face. This interruption in Qi flow can also lead to facial deviation.

In such cases, a formula that unblocks the meridians and disperses Wind is often effective, just one dose can bring complete recovery. This type of condition is entirely different from hemiplegia and cannot be treated with the same formulas used for that disorder.

Differentiating Drooling from Phlegm-Fluids

Some have asked: "Isn't the liquid drooling from the corners of the mouth a form of phlegm-fluid?"

I replied: "I've treated this condition many times, and in every case, what flowed was clear, thin saliva, not thick phlegm. It's clearly a case of Qi deficiency failing to secure body fluids.

If this is hard to believe, just observe: eight or nine out of ten children drool when their Qi is not yet fully developed, and two or three out of ten elderly people drool when their Qi has become weak. Cross-reference this with other symptoms, and it is beyond doubt, drooling results from Qi deficiency, not from phlegm."

Differentiating Dry Stool from Wind and Fire

Some have asked: "In cases of hemiplegia accompanied by dry stool, the ancients called it 'Wind Dryness,' suggesting the presence of both Wind and Fire. Does that make sense?"

I replied: "If the condition were truly caused by Wind and Fire, then dispersing Wind, clearing Fire, moistening dryness, and promoting bowel movement should resolve the issue. Once the bowels move, the Wind is dispersed, the Fire is cleared, and the dryness should naturally disappear.

Yet in practice, I have often seen patients treated with purgative formulas, only for their stools to become even drier afterward. These treatments fail because they overlook a basic truth: normal bowel movements do not occur by passive flow through the intestines, they require effort.

If a patient with hemiplegia lacks the strength to move their limbs or speak with the tongue, how can they possibly generate the strength needed in the lower body to push stool downward?

By this reasoning, the cause is not Wind and Fire, but a lack of Qi, insufficient strength to propel the bowels. When stool remains in the large intestine for extended periods without being discharged, it naturally dries out over time."

Differentiating Polyuria, Enuresis, and Incontinence

Differentiating Frequent Urination, Enuresis, and Incontinence

Some people ask: "Frequent urination, enuresis, and urinary incontinence, are they caused by Fire or by deficiency? Is there a meaningful distinction?"

I reply: If there is pain in the penis during urination, with urine dripping out in small amounts and appearing reddish, this is a sign of internal Fire.

If the patient is elderly or constitutionally weak, and the urination is prolonged, mildly painful, and the urine is pale and clear, then it is a case of Qi deficiency.

When the urethral opening relaxes and urine flows out without the person being aware of it, this is called enuresis.

When the person feels the urge to urinate and consciously tries to hold it, but urine still flows out involuntarily, this is urinary incontinence.

These patterns describe conditions that arise from dysfunction within the urinary system itself.

However, if frequent urination, enuresis, or incontinence occur in the context of hemiplegia, there is no pain in the penis. In such cases, the root issue is Qi deficiency, the body lacks the strength to contain and lift the bladder's contents.

Differentiating Slurred Speech

Differentiating Slurred Speech as Not Caused by Phlegm and Fire

Some people have asked, "When a person can't speak clearly, it has traditionally been explained as slurred speech caused by phlegm and fire obstructing the root of the tongue. Does that explanation make sense?"

I replied, "No, it's not caused by phlegm or fire. The tongue contains two internal channels that connect to the brain. These function like airways for the body's vital energy and allow the tongue to move so that speech is possible.

When one side of the body loses its energy, as in hemiplegia, that side becomes immobile. The same thing happens to the corresponding half of the tongue, it also lacks energy and cannot move fully. As a result, speech becomes slurred or unclear.

You can observe the same pattern in children who haven't developed enough energy to walk; they often speak unclearly.

Similarly, elderly people with weak vitality also tend to have slurred or indistinct speech. This proves that the root cause is a lack of vital energy, not phlegm or fire."

Differentiating Jaw Clenching and Teeth Grinding

Some have asked: "If hemiplegia isn't caused by Wind or Fire, then why do some patients clench their jaws or grind their teeth?"

I replied: "Jaw clenching and teeth grinding are two entirely different phenomena. The ancients mistakenly lumped them together as one symptom, a sign of careless clinical observation.

Jaw clenching is a deficiency pattern, while teeth grinding is an excess pattern.

In jaw clenching, the mouth is tightly shut and cannot be opened.

In teeth grinding, the teeth grind against each other audibly, producing a distinct sound.

In conditions like Cold Damage, epidemic illness, miscellaneous diseases, and gynecological disorders, both types can be seen, some patients with deficient Qi exhibit jaw clenching, and others with excess conditions show teeth grinding.

However, in cases of hemiplegia, you may see jaw clenching, but **never** teeth grinding. In some instances, the clenching is so severe that the lower teeth get pressed inward, producing a rasping or grinding sound. This may resemble teeth grinding, but it is not. It remains a deficiency pattern.

If a patient has no hemiplegia and no other obvious illness, and suddenly develops jaw clenching, the likely cause is Wind obstructing the meridians and preventing Qi from reaching the upper body. In such cases, a formula that unblocks the meridians can bring rapid recovery."

Early Signs Before Onset of the Disease

Some have asked: "After Yuan Qi (vital energy) begins to decline, but before hemiplegia appears, are there any recognizable signs of deficiency?"

I have treated this condition more than any other in my lifetime and understand it in the greatest detail. Each time I treated a patient and they recovered, I would ask about any symptoms they experienced prior to the onset of hemiplegia. Their answers revealed consistent patterns.

Some reported occasional bouts of dizziness; others described unexplained heaviness in the head. Some heard wind-like sounds in their ears, while others heard a buzzing like cicadas. Some experienced prolonged twitching of the lower eyelid, and some noticed that one eye gradually became smaller.

Some said their eyes would occasionally appear dazed or unfocused without reason. Others reported seeing whirlwinds or swirls of light in their vision for extended periods. Some felt cold air lingering in their nose. A few had intermittent twitching of the upper lip, or a sensation of the lips drawing tightly together.

Some drooled during sleep. Some, once mentally sharp, suddenly experienced memory lapses. Others found themselves speaking less, trailing off mid-sentence, or speaking incoherently. Some had unexplained episodes of wheezing.

There were cases of persistent trembling in one hand, or both hands. Some reported that their ring finger would sometimes fail to straighten. Others noticed their thumb moving involuntarily. Some experienced numbness in the arms or legs without cause, or spontaneous muscle twitching.

Several said they felt waves of cold air rising from beneath their fingernails or toenails, or from the gaps around their knees. Some described sudden weakness in the ankles, causing the feet to collapse outward. Others reported leg or toe cramps without warning. Some felt as if their legs were entangled while walking, like garlic being mashed in a mortar.

Still others experienced chest tightness, shortness of breath, or sudden rapid heartbeat. A few reported episodes of unexplained stiffness in the neck. Some felt their bodies sinking into the bed during sleep.

All of these are signs of gradually weakening vital energy. But because there is no pain or itch, no fever or chills, and no interference with appetite or daily function, these signs are the easiest to overlook.

On Pediatric Hemiplegia

Some have asked, "Can children also suffer from hemiplegia?"

I reply: "Yes, children can develop this condition anytime from infancy, around one year old, through early childhood. It is uncommon for a child to develop hemiplegia suddenly. More often, it appears after illnesses such as cold damage (typhoid-like febrile diseases), epidemics, pox, or severe vomiting and diarrhea.

In these cases, the child's vital energy (Qi) gradually becomes depleted during recovery. The complexion turns pale or bluish-white, and over time, the child loses the ability to move their hands and feet. Some even develop convulsions or muscle spasms. The entire body may become limp, as if made of clay, because Qi can no longer circulate to the limbs.

Ancient physicians often misclassified this as a Wind disorder, but this was likely due to their limited experience in treating pediatric hemiplegia."

On Paralysis

Some have asked: "You've explained that when vital Qi (Yuan Qi) collapses into the left or right side of the body, it results in hemiplegia. Can it also collapse into the upper or lower half of the body?"

I replied: "When a person loses 50% of their vital energy and the remaining half continues to circulate through the body, signs of Qi deficiency will certainly emerge. But if the remaining Qi suddenly collapses into the upper body and can no longer descend, the result is paralysis of both legs.

Yet according to traditional theories, this condition, classified as *wei* syndrome (atrophy disorder), is said to arise from damp-heat in the Stomach channel of the Foot

Yangming, which rises and 'steams' the Lungs. The heat scorches the lung lobes, the skin and hair become withered, and atrophy follows. Treatments based on that theory typically use cold and purgative formulas to clear heat and eliminate dampness.

In my view, those formulas may be appropriate for treating damp-heat *bi* syndrome (painful obstruction of the legs), but they are unsuitable for *wei* syndrome. Why? Because when leg paralysis results from *bi* syndrome, pain is always present, before and after paralysis. But in *wei* syndrome, the legs suddenly become immobile without any pain from beginning to end.

If one fails to distinguish between superficial signs and the root cause, or confuses deficiency with excess, how can future practitioners avoid being misled and causing harm?"

Bu Yang Huan Wu Tang

Bu Yang Huan Wu Tang (Yang Restoration for the Lost Half Decoction)

This formula is used to treat hemiplegia, facial asymmetry (drooping of the mouth and eyes), slurred speech, drooling, dry stools, frequent urination, enuresis, and urinary incontinence.

Ingredients

Pin Yin	Latin Name	English Name	Amount (grams)
Huang Qi	Astragali Radix	Astragalus Root	120
(Dang) Gui Wei	Angelicae Sinensis Extremitas Radix	Angelica Root Tail	6
Chi Shao	Paeoniae Radix Rubra	Red Peony Root	3
Di Long	Pheretima	Earthworm	3
Chuan Xiong	Chuanxiong Rhizoma	Cnidium	3
Tao Ren	Persicae Semen (mashed)	Peach Kernel (mashed)	3
Hong Hua	Carthemi Flos	Safflower	3

Huang Qi (raw) 120g, Dang Gui Wei 6g, Chi Shao 4.5g, Di Long 3g, Chuan Xiong 3g, Tao Ren 3g, Hong Hua 3g

Preparation and Usage

Boil with water together and drink the decoction

At the early stage of hemiplegia, when the condition has just appeared, add 3 grams of *Fang Feng* (Saposhnikovia Root) to the formula. After taking four or five doses, *Fang Feng* should no longer be included.

If the patient has heard from others and is fearful of taking large amounts of *Huang Qi* (Astragalus Root), we may need to accommodate this by starting with 30–60 grams, then gradually increasing to 120 grams. Once the formula begins to show effect, increase to two doses per day, amounting to 240 grams of *Huang Qi* daily. After five or six days of this, reduce to one dose per day.

For those who have been ill for two to three months and were previously treated with overly cooling herbs based on classical prescriptions, add 12–15 grams of *Fu Zi* (Aconite Root) to warm and restore Yang. If the patient was given too many Wind-dispersing herbs, add 12–15 grams of *Dang Shen* (Codonopsis) to support Qi. If no Wind-dispersing herbs were used, this addition is unnecessary.

Though this is an excellent therapeutic formula, it may not fully reverse advanced cases where Yuan Qi is severely depleted, such as when the shoulder has sunken by two to three finger-widths, the arm is contracted and cannot be extended, the ankles collapse outward, or the patient has lost all ability to speak. These cases are not curable. However, regular use of the formula can still help stabilize the condition and prevent further deterioration.

After recovery with this formula, treatment should not be stopped abruptly. The patient should continue taking one dose every three to five days, or at least once every seven to eight days. Discontinuing completely may lead to a relapse or even the development of Qi collapse in the future.

As for the *Huang Qi* (Astragalus Root) in this formula, it is effective regardless of where it is grown, its medicinal strength is consistent and suitable for use in all cases.

Formula Rhyme

Chi Shao and Chuan Xiong stir Blood's flow,

Gui Wei with Di Long make channels grow.

One hundred twenty grams of Huang Qi leads,

Tao Ren and Hong Hua clear stasis with speed.

On Plague Vomiting, Diarrhea, and Muscle Spasms

The illness characterized by vomiting, diarrhea, and muscle spasms was traditionally called Cholera (Huo Luan). During the Song Dynasty, the Imperial Hospital formulated a remedy that became the official prescription: Huo Xiang Zheng Qi San (Agastache Powder to Rectify the Qi). But to treat a condition caused by external evil harming the body's righteous energy with a formula that instead disperses and attacks that very righteous energy, doesn't this bring shame to the name of great physicians?

In the first year of the Daoguang reign (1821, the year of Xinsi), a plague spread across several provinces, bringing widespread cases of vomiting, diarrhea, and spasms. The situation in the capital was even more severe, with a high death toll. So many people died that the poor could not afford burials, and the government had to distribute funds and coffins. In just over a month, more than hundreds of thousands of taels of gold were spent.

At the time, some physicians treated patients successfully with warming herbs such as ginseng, white atractylodes, dried ginger, and aconite, and concluded that the illness was a cold-type disorder. Others treated with cooling herbs such as scutellaria, coptis, gardenia, and phellodendron, and concluded it was a fire-toxic condition.

I said, "That's not correct. Regardless of gender or age, everyone was suffering from the same disease, plague (wen du)." Some responded, "If it's the same disease, how can both hot herbs like dried ginger and aconite, and cold herbs like scutellaria and coptis, be effective?"

I replied, "Cooling herbs like scutellaria and coptis were effective at the onset, when the patient was still strong and the toxic force was dominant. Warming herbs like dried ginger and aconite were effective in the later stages, after the toxin had weakened but the patient had become depleted and their vital energy was failing."

Some asked again, "There were patients who took Huang Qin (Scutellaria), Huang Lian (Coptis), Gan Jiang (Dried Ginger), and Fu Zi (Aconite) without any effect, in fact, they got worse. Why?"

I replied, "Observe those who recovered after being treated with bloodletting. The blood that came out was dark purple or black, wasn't that the result of toxic heat from the plague burning the blood? Plague toxins enter through the mouth and nose, first invading the airways, then spreading into the bloodstream. This causes the Qi and Blood to coagulate, blocking the body's fluid pathways so that water cannot be discharged, leading to vomiting and diarrhea.

At the onset of the illness, if you lance the blood vessels at the crook of the elbow, the blood that comes out will be dark and thick. When this toxic blood is released, the patient often recovers. Some asked me, 'What acupuncture point should we prick? Please be specific.' I said, 'Though I'm skilled at acupuncture, there's no need to debate, it's the point called Chize (LU5). The respiratory and circulatory systems run throughout the body, and there are four or five blood vessels around Chize on both the left and right arms. Pricking any of them will produce blood and can help cure the disease.

Even points slightly above or below Chize can be used effectively.'

In short, bloodletting works for excess conditions caused by wind and fire. But in deficiency conditions, it only makes things worse. This is a truth many acupuncturists know but hesitate to admit. Still, in urgent cases, bloodletting is quick and convenient, which is why it is often used."

While performing acupuncture, simultaneously use Detoxifying and Blood-Activating Decoction (Jie Du Huo Xue Tang) to move the blood and clear the poison. In such cases, recovery often follows after just one dose. However, this illness progresses extremely rapidly and consumes vital energy at an alarming rate. It can become life-threatening within a day, or even half a day.

If vomiting and diarrhea continue for just a couple of hours, and leg cramps appear, it indicates Qi deficiency in the legs. If arm cramps appear, it means Qi is depleted in the arms. If you see sunken eyelids, profuse sweating like running water, and limbs that are cold as ice, then even mentioning the harm of cold-natured herbs is unnecessary. At this stage, even my Detoxifying and Blood-Activating Decoction, which I formulated myself, would no longer help and might even worsen the situation.

At such a critical moment, regardless of how dry the tongue and mouth are, or how intense the thirst is, even if the patient drinks several bowls of cold water, do not hesitate to use Emergency Yang-Restoring Decoction (Ji Jiu Hui Yang Tang), based on Dried Ginger (Gan Jiang) and Aconite (Fu Zi). One dose can pull the patient back from the brink of death.

This life-saving method is not something that shallow or inexperienced physicians are likely to understand.

Jie Du Huo Xue Tang

Jie Du Huo Xue Tang (Detoxing and Blood-circulating Decoction)

Ingredients

Pin Yin	Latin Name	English Name	Amount (grams)
Lian Qiao	Forsythiae Fructus	Forsythia Fruit	6
Ge Gen	Puerariae Radix	Kudzu Root	6
Chai Hu	Bupleuri Radix	Hare's Ear Root	9
Dang Gui	Angelicae Sinensis Radix	Angelica Root	6
Sheng Di Huang	Rehmanniae Radix	Rehmanniae Root	15
Chi Shao	Paeoniae Radix Rubra	Red Peony Root	9

Pin Yin	Latin Name	English Name	Amount (grams)
Tao Ren	Persicae Semen (mashed)	Peach Kernel (mashed)	24
Hong Hua	Carthemi Flos	Safflower	15
Zhi Ke	Aurantii Fructus	Bitter Orange	3
Gan Cao	Glycyrrhizae Radix	Licorice Root	6

Lian Qiao 6g, Ge Gen 6g, Chai Hu 9g, Dang Gui 6g, Sheng Di Huang 15g, Chi Shao 9g, Tao Ren (mashed) 24g, Hong Hua 15g, Zhi Ke 3g, Gan Cao 6g

Boil together with water and drink the decoction

Formula Rhyme

Lian Qiao and Tao Ren purge the strain,

Hong Hua, Zhi Qiao, Ge Gen remain.

Chi Shao, Sheng Di, Dang Gui too,

Chai Hu and Gan Cao see you through.

Boil in water—gently restore,

For early-stage vomit and diarrhea's uproar.

This formula is intended for vomiting and diarrhea in the early stage of the illness. If symptoms such as profuse sweating, cold limbs, and sunken eyelids appear, it should no longer be used.

Ji Jiu Hui Yang Tang

Ji Jiu Hui Yang Tang (Emergency Yang Reviving Decoction)

If vomiting and diarrhea are accompanied by spasms, chills, and profuse sweating, this formula must be used. Do not hesitate to administer it, even if the patient has intense thirst and drinks large amounts of cold water.

Ingredients

Pin Yin	Latin Name	English Name	Amount (grams)
Dang Shen	Codonopsis Radix	Codonopsis	24

Pin Yin	Latin Name	English Name	Amount (grams)
(Zhi) Fu Zi	Aconiti Radix Lateralis Preparata	Aconite Accessory Root	24
Gan Jiang	Zingiberis Rhizoma	Dried Ginger	12
Bai Zhu	Atractylodis Macrocephalae Rhizoma	White Atractylodes	12
Gan Cao	Glycyrrhizae Radix	Licorice Root	9
Tao Ren	Persicae Semen (mashed)	Peach Kernel (mashed)	6
Hong Hua	Carthemi Flos	Safflower	6

Dang Shen 24g, Fu Zi 24g, Gan Jiang 12g, Bai Zhu 12g, Gan Cao 9g, Tao Ren (mashed) 6g, Hong Hua 6g

Formula Rhyme

Ren Shen, Fu Zi, Gan Jiang warm,

Zhu, Cao, Tao, and Hong transform.

With courage clear and vision true,

This blend revives and pulls you through.

Though Tao and Hong move Blood with might,

They stir no harm when Yang takes flight.

If you clearly distinguish the boundaries between *Jie Du Huo Xue Tang* (Detoxifying and Blood-Activating Decoction) and *Ji Jiu Hui Yang Tang* (Emergency Yang-Restoring Decoction), there will be no case that cannot be effectively treated. Take heed! Take heed!

On Pediatric Convulsions Are Not Caused by Wind

The treatment of convulsions is often ineffective today, not because modern doctors are treating it incorrectly, but because they've been misled by traditional formulas. The problem lies not only in the old prescriptions, but also in the theories and naming conventions handed down. For example, the condition was labeled as "Wind Convulsion," and the character **wind** (风) is particularly misleading.

Since this condition often arises after illnesses such as typhoid (cold damage), epidemic fevers, pox, or prolonged vomiting and diarrhea, ancient physicians called it *Slow Wind Shock* (慢惊风). But using these three characters together as a diagnostic term is not only linguistically absurd, it also reflects a lack of careful observation of the true origin of the disease.

If it were truly caused by Wind, then Wind would have had to enter through the skin into the meridians, and there should be clear exterior-to-interior symptoms we can observe. But that's not what actually happens.

If there are no signs of external invasion, why did ancient authors and physicians so often claim this disease was caused by Wind? It's because, during an attack, they observed the neck and back arching rigidly backward, the eyes rolling upward in a daze, the jaw clenching shut, drooling and foaming at the mouth, a rattling sound in the throat, and unconsciousness, and they concluded it must be Wind stroke.

But what they failed to understand was this: the arching of the neck and spine, the twitching limbs, and the clenched hands and feet are all signs that the vital energy is too weak to hold the body together. The upturned eyes and locked jaw result from Qi deficiency that cannot rise to the head. The drooling occurs because Qi is too weak to hold the fluids in place. And the rattling sound in the throat is not due to actual phlegm, but to deficient Qi unable to return to its source.

If this principle isn't understood, observe elderly individuals nearing the end of life after prolonged illness. You'll often see a stiff neck, a heavy and unresponsive body, eyes fixed and staring, tightly clenched teeth, drooling, a rapid sawing-like sound from the throat, or cold sweat covering the entire body, all of which clearly reveal the signs of depleted vital Qi.

Now compare these with the symptoms of convulsions: eyes rolling upward, locked jaw, drooling, and the same harsh, sawing-like breathing sound. The resemblance is unmistakable, convulsions are undoubtedly rooted in Qi deficiency. When the vital Qi is empty, it can no longer circulate to the blood vessels. Without Qi to move the blood, stasis inevitably occurs.

So how can it be appropriate to treat a condition of Qi deficiency and blood stasis with formulas that scatter wind and clear heat? It is unquestionably a mistaken approach.

When wind-dispersing formulas are used in the absence of wind, they disperse the body's vital Qi. When fire-clearing formulas are given without actual fire, they cause the blood to congeal. If, on top of that, attacking, purging, and depleting formulas are used, the result is scattered Qi and stagnant blood, how can survival be expected?

If we trace the root cause, these patients did not die at the hands of the doctors who treated them, but at the hands of those who wrote the books that misled them.

Whenever I meet seasoned pediatric practitioners, they never delay or mislead in treating patients. They know that the classical formulas for convulsions are ineffective, so when they encounter such cases, they often refrain from intervention.

And yet, there are also true experts who can foresee the onset of convulsions based on a child's current symptoms. Even though no effective classical formula exists, they still inform the family that convulsions are likely to occur in the future. How can they be so sure?

Before the onset of convulsions, there are always early warning signs. These include: a sunken fontanelle, lethargy with eyes open during sleep, tongue trembling inside the mouth, inability to cry, crying without tears, flaring nostrils, rattling phlegm in the throat, difficulty lifting the head, clenched jaw with silence, icy cold limbs, foaming at the mouth, a bulging chest like an inverted bowl, rapid and labored breathing, pale or bluish complexion, profuse sweating like running water, inability to nurse, greenish stool, audible bowel sounds, simultaneous diarrhea and coughing, and twitching muscles. These are all pre-convulsive symptoms.

You don't need to see all twenty signs, just one or two is enough to predict that convulsions are likely to occur. Among these cases, some can be cured, and others cannot. The treatments and formulas for each will be detailed below.

For instance, if the child has wide, dazed eyes, refuses food, does not cry, and makes phlegmy, wheezing sounds while breathing, although the condition is serious, it is still treatable.

However, if the forehead turns gray, the testicles are tightly retracted upward, or the pulse is extremely thin or absent, then even if the outward appearance seems mild, the prognosis is unfortunately beyond cure.

Ke Bao Sheng Su Tang

Ke Bao Sheng Su Tang (Child Life Saving and Reviving Decoction)

This formula is effective for children who develop twitching limbs, backward arching of the neck and spine, upturned and dazed eyes, clenched jaws, drooling, lethargy, and unconsciousness as a result of prolonged illness following cold damage (such as typhoid fever), epidemic infections, pox, or persistent vomiting and diarrheal, all of which lead to depletion of vital Qi.

Ingredients

Pin Yin	Latin Name	English Name	Amount (grams)
Huang Qi	Astragali Radix	Astragalus Root	45
Dang Shen	Codonopsis Radix	Codonopsis	9

Medical Forest Error Corrections

Pin Yin	Latin Name	English Name	Amount (grams)
Bai Zhu	Atractylodis Macrocephalae Rhizoma	White Atractylodes	6
Gan Cao	Glycyrrhizae Radix	Licorice Root	6
Dang Gui	Angelicae Sinensis Radix	Angelica Root	6
Bai Shao	Paeoniae Radix Alba	White Peony Root	6
Suan Zao Ren	Ziziphi Spinosae Semen	Sour Jujube Seed	9
Shan Zhu Yu	Corni Fructus	Asiatic Cornelian Cherry Fruit	3
Gou Qi Zi	Lycii Fructus	Chinese Wolfberry	6
Bu Gu Zhi	Psoraleae Fructus	Psoraleae Fruit	3
He Tao	Juglandis Semen	Walnut	1 whole

Huang Qi (raw) 45g, Dang Shen 9g, Bai Zhu 6g, Gan Cao 6g, Dang Gui 6g, Bai Shao 6g, Suan Zao Ren 9g, Shan Zhu Yu 3g, Gou Qi Zi 6g, Gu Zhi 3g, He Tao (with shell, broken) 1 piece

Preparation and Usage

Boil them together with water and drink the decoction

The listed dosage for this formula is intended for a four-year-old child. For a two-year-old, reduce the dosage by half. For a one-year-old, use one-third. For an infant of two to three months, use one-quarter of the dose. There is no need to rigidly limit the number of doses. In my experience treating this condition, children often needed two to three doses in a single day. The formula should be continued until convulsions stop. It is essential to inform the child's family not to discontinue the medicine just because the convulsions have ceased. A few additional doses should still be taken to fully restore the vital Qi.

Formula Rhyme

Gu Zhi, Suan Zao calm and tone,

Zhu, Gui, Shao Yao firm the bone.

Ren Shen, Huang Qi, Gan Cao blend,

Shan Yu, Gou Qi nourish and mend.

Boil in water, then don't omit,

One whole walnut, shell and all, ground to grit.

On Pox is not Fetal Toxin

Pediatric pox has been written about since the Han Dynasty, with countless physicians authoring books and formulating prescriptions over the centuries. Yet most simply categorized the disease into "favorable," "critical," and "unfavorable" types to judge its severity and the likelihood of survival or death, without ever explaining the true cause of the illness.

As a result, later generations took different paths: some followed *Bao Yuan Tang* (Preserve the Vital Qi Decoction), using Huang Qi (Astragalus Root) and Ren Shen (Ginseng); some followed *Gui Zong Tang* (Returning to the Origin Decoction), using Da Huang (Rhubarb) and Shi Gao (Gypsum); and others used *Jie Du Tang* (Detoxification Decoction), featuring Xi Jiao (Rhinoceros Horn) and Huang Lian (Coptis).

It was the same disease, yet the treatment varied widely.

For cases of *favorable* or *critical* pox, if the child's condition is assessed carefully, whether strong or weak, then choosing to supplement, purge, clear, or cool accordingly can still lead to recovery.

But when faced with *unfavorable* pox, there are no prescriptions offered. Instead, people simply blame fate, because they do not understand the real cause of the disease.

Some ask, "If the ancients didn't understand the true cause of pox, then how could they predict, upon seeing unfavorable pox, exactly how many days the patient had left to live?"

I replied, "That's not because they understood the root cause of the disease. It's because they had observed countless pox cases and, through experience, knew the timing of the disease's progression: on which day the pustules would appear, what form or color they would take, and what symptoms would arise on each day. And when none of the treatments worked, they knew on which day the patient would die. That's how they made such predictions, not through understanding, but through repeated observation.

If they had truly known the underlying cause of pox, how could there have been no effective formula to treat it?"

Then some asked, "Based on what you've said, is there a way to save a patient with unfavorable pox?"

I said: "Critical-stage pox can be readily treated, there's no need for much discussion. As for the most severe, life-threatening cases, the so-called 'unfavorable pox', they each have identifiable causes. Once those causes are properly understood and differentiated, how could recovery not be possible?

Take the cases I've treated: the pox was trapped inside and couldn't break through the surface. The whole body was covered in dense clusters, as fine as silkworm casings, as flat and tight as snake skin. In some, the pox erupted before any fever appeared. The lesions were purple-black, packed across the body with no gaps, or appeared in alternating patches of purple, white, and gray. The head was buried in pox, the mouth sealed shut. The neck was locked, the cheeks held tight. There was no swelling, but fluid-filled blisters covered the skin. The rashes were flat, without pus or crusting.

After the rash appeared, the child suffered constant convulsions. Bright red blood streamed from all nine orifices. The cough was hoarse and weak, and they choked whenever trying to drink water. By days six or seven, the itching became unbearable, yet when the rashes were scratched open, no blood emerged. By days seven or eight, diarrhea began, and appetite disappeared. At the peak of danger, they could not lift their head, the feet were distorted, the eyes rolled upward, and the neck and spine arched backwards.

Even in cases like these, once such symptoms appear, if one can clearly differentiate between deficiency and excess, the patient still has a chance to survive."

Those who truly understand this recognize that I am filling in the gaps left by the ancients and offering real solutions for the difficult cases we face today. But those who do not grasp this truth make baseless criticisms, accusing me of arrogance, unaware that it is not arrogance, but insight into the true cause of pox. Unlike others who merely echo inherited theories, I do not claim, as many schools do, that pox always results from so-called fetal toxins.

Various books claim that smallpox did not exist before the Han Dynasty. But if it is said to be caused by fetal toxins, are we to assume that people before the Han Dynasty were not born of parents? That would be the most absurd claim of all.

Some ancient theories suggest that fetal toxins are hidden in the internal organs, yet before the onset of pox, why are the organs entirely healthy? Others claim that the toxins are stored in the muscles, yet why do no sores appear on the skin before the pox erupts? Still others say the toxins are buried in the bone marrow and are triggered by fright, falls, indigestion, or exposure to cold, leading to the development of smallpox.

But if such minor incidents can indeed trigger smallpox, then the fault lies with the person's own carelessness. However, if you carefully observe periods when smallpox outbreaks are widespread, not just a few isolated cases but affecting entire regions or even multiple provinces at once, can we really believe that so many people were all "careless" at the same time? Clearly, that explanation is even more unreasonable.

Look at the doctors who perform vaccination today, regardless of how many children they inoculate, every case results in a favorable form of pox. But if smallpox were truly caused by fetal toxins, wouldn't there naturally be variations in the severity of those toxins? Those with heavier toxins should develop critical or unfavorable pox. So how is it that all vaccinated cases are favorable? If you consider this carefully, you'll see that the theory of "fetal toxins" is far from unshakable.

What people fail to understand is that smallpox is not caused by fetal toxins, but by turbid Qi carried in the fetal blood. A fetus begins with a drop of pure essence and gradually develops its internal organs and limbs entirely from the mother's blood. The turbid Qi present in that maternal-fetal blood remains hidden in the body's nourishing blood after birth. When a seasonal epidemic arises that stirs up this internal turbidity, the pathogen enters through the nose and mouth, travels along the respiratory tract into the blood vessels, and forces the turbid Qi outward through the skin.

The eruption appears red like flowers, hence the name *Heavenly Flowers* (Tian Hua, or smallpox). The shape is round like beans, thus it is also called *Dou* (pox).

In short, when a person contracts a mild plague, the toxin is expelled along with the pox eruption, this results in a *favorable pox*. When the plague is more severe, the toxin lingers within the body and cannot be fully released through the skin, leading to a *critical pox*. And when the infection is at its most severe, the toxin scorches the blood from within. This internal burning causes the blood to congeal, congealed blood turns purple, while dead blood turns black. Thus, purple-black pox lesions are a hallmark of severe cases.

When dead blood obstructs circulation, the toxin can no longer exit through the skin and is instead driven inward to attack the internal organs. The viscera are then tormented by toxic fire, giving rise to a host of reversal patterns involving the organs.

This is precisely what traditional smallpox texts refer to as "unfavorable pox of a particular meridian." But in truth, it is not that a particular meridian has produced an unfavorable pox, it is that the meridian in question has been afflicted by plague toxin.

Whether a case of pox is favorable or unfavorable depends entirely on the severity of the plague. The key to treating pox lies in the method used to expel the plague toxin. If the toxin is not eliminated, even a mild rash will inevitably lead to death. But if the toxin is successfully removed, even a heavy eruption will not endanger life.

Medical texts on pox speak only of treating "fetal toxin," without recognizing the need to address the plague toxin. And even when they do acknowledge the plague toxin, they fail to understand that its nesting ground is in the blood.

If one can accurately assess the intensity of the plague toxin, determine whether blood circulation is flowing smoothly or obstructed, and distinguish between deficiency and excess of vital Qi, then treating unfavorable pox and saving lives becomes as easy as turning over the palm of your hand.

This is what it means to understand the root, just one sentence will reveal everything.

On Pox Fluid: Not a Transformation of Blood

When pox first appears, it is red. After five or six days, it turns into a clear fluid, then becomes a white fluid, followed by a turbid fluid, then yellow pus, and finally forms a scab. The ancients often claimed that the fluid in pox was transformed from blood. But if that were true, red blood would have to be able to turn white. Let's test this idea with a cup of blood: whether you treat it with alum or boil it over fire, can you make it turn into clear liquid, white fluid, turbid fluid, or yellow pus?

In truth, pox arises from turbid Qi trapped in the blood within the vessels. When an epidemic toxin triggers this internal turbidity, it enters through the mouth and nose, passes through the respiratory tract, and reaches the bloodstream. There, it drives the turbid Qi, along with some blood and fluids from the airways, out through the skin and pores, forming the round red appearance of pox.

116

After five or six days, the blood originally present in the pox returns to the blood vessels, leaving behind only turbid Qi and body fluids. These remaining fluids are transparent and thus called "clear fluid." As this clear fluid is simmered by the epidemic toxin, it thickens and turns white, becoming "white fluid." Continued heating turns this into a denser, murkier substance, "turbid fluid." With further progression, the turbid fluid thickens into something resembling pus and becomes "yellow pus." Eventually, this yellow pus dries and scabs over.

If no fluid appears in a pox lesion, it is because the blood failed to return to the vessels. This failure is usually due to the epidemic toxin heating and congealing the blood within the vessels, blocking normal circulation. If the blood stasis is cleared and circulation is restored, there is no reason to fear that the pox will fail to produce fluid.

On Choking When Drinking Water

On Choking When Drinking Water During a Pox Outbreak

After four or five days, or sometimes seven or eight days, into a pox outbreak, some patients begin to choke whenever they drink water. The ancients attributed this to toxic fire accumulating in the throat and classified it as an incurable condition.

It is because they do not understand the anatomical structure of the throat, specifically, the left and right air passages. Behind the tongue lies the larynx, which connects to the lungs. Behind the larynx is the pharynx, which leads to the stomach. At the junction between the front of the pharynx and the back of the larynx, there are two recessed channels called the left and right Qi gates.

At the root of the tongue is a thin white flap, about the thickness of a coin, called the epiglottis. It normally covers the entrance to the lung passage and the two air gates. When we swallow food or drink, the tip of the tongue presses against the roof of the mouth, guiding the epiglottis to seal the airway tightly. This ensures that food or drink bypasses the lung passage and enters the esophagus behind it.

Observe someone eating: if food has just entered the throat but hasn't yet reached the esophagus, and the person suddenly laughs, the upward surge of air may pop open the epiglottis. A grain of rice or a drop of water may then slip into one of the airways and be immediately expelled through the nose, this serves as proof of the mechanism.

Now, during a pox outbreak, plague toxins scorch the epiglottis. When blood congeals there, the epiglottis can no longer close the airways tightly. Water then seeps through and causes choking. Food, being more solid, does not seep in as easily through a small gap, so it doesn't usually trigger choking. Once the congealed blood in the epiglottis is cleared, the choking stops immediately.

On Itch After Seven to Eight Days of Pox

To understand the cause of itching in pox, one must first clearly distinguish between *pi* and *fu*, the dermis and epidermis. *Pi* refers to the dermis, and *fu* refers to the epidermis. Without differentiating the two, how can one understand why pox itches? For example, when someone is scalded by hot soup or burned by fire, a blister will form. The thin layer, like paper, is the *fu* (epidermis); beneath it, between the *fu* and the flesh, lies the thicker *pi* (dermis).

At around six or seven days after the pox erupts, the plague toxin, turbid Qi, and bodily fluids are lodged between the outer dermis (*pi*) and inner epidermis (*fu*). Within the "nest" of the pox, the body's righteous Qi is too weak to reach the lesions and complete the processes of fluid transformation, suppuration, and scabbing. As a result, the toxin cannot be expelled outward through the *fu*, nor can it be drawn inward through the *pi*. Trapped between the dermis and epidermis, the toxin causes intense itching.

Many physicians follow the statement in the *Su Wen* that "all sores and itching belong to fire," and thus resort to cold and clearing herbs that suppress vital Qi. This not only fails to relieve the itching but also injures the Stomach Qi. Others focus solely on Qi-tonifying herbs, but the more they supplement Qi, the more blood stasis accumulates. The more stagnant the blood, the harder it becomes for Qi to reach the surface of the skin.

At this point, formulas that both tonify Qi and break up blood stasis should be used to clear the channels of blood circulation. When Qi can reach the skin directly, the itching always stops, often with just a single dose.

Tong Jing Zhu Yu Tang

Tong Jing Zhu Yu Tang (Channel Opening and Blood Stasis Expelling Decoction)

This formula is suitable regardless of the presentation of the pox, whether the lesions are clustered, hood-shaped, pot-lid shaped, finely scattered across the body, a mix of papules and rashes, or manifest as floating blisters; whether their color is purple, dusky, or black; and whether the accompanying symptoms include dry retching, restlessness, or inability to sleep day or night. In all such cases, especially with unfavorable pox, the underlying cause is blood stasis obstructing the vessels.

The medicinal nature of this formula is neither overly cold nor overly hot, neither overly attacking nor overly purging. It strikes a perfect balance. Truly, this is an excellent prescription.

Ingredients

Pin Yin	Latin Name	English Name	Amount (grams)
Tao Ren	Persicae Semen (mashed)	Peach Kernel (mashed)	24
Hong Hua	Carthemi Flos	Safflower	12

Pin Yin	Latin Name	English Name	Amount (grams)
Chi Shao	Paeoniae Radix Rubra	Red Peony Root	9
Chuan Shan Jia	Squama Manitis	Pangolin Scales	12
Zao Jiao Ci	Spina Gleditsiae	Chinese Honey Locust Spine	18
Lian Qiao	Forsythiae Fructus	Forsythia Fruit	9
Di Long	Pheretima	Earthworm	9
Chai Hu	Bupleuri Radix	Hare's Ear Root	3
She Xiang	Moschus	Musk	0.15

Tao Ren 24g, Hong Hua 12g, Chi Shao 9g, Shan Jia 12g, Zao Ci 18g, Lian Qiao (without) 9g, Di Long 9g, Chai Hu 3g, She Xiang 3 Li (wrap in silk)

Preparation and Usage

Boil together with water to drink the decoction

If the stool is dry, add 6 grams of Da Huang (Rhubarb Root), and discontinue it once the bowel movement becomes smooth. Around the fifth or sixth day, when clear fluid or white fluid appears in the pox, discontinue She Xiang (Musk), add 15 grams of Huang Qi (Astragalus Root), and reduce both Chuan Shan Jia (Pangolin Scales) and Zao Jiao Ci (Chinese Honey Locust Spine) by half.

By the seventh or eighth day, reduce the doses of Tao Ren (Peach Kernel) and Hong Hua (Safflower) by half as well, and Huang Qi may be increased to 24 grams.

This formula is designed for a child aged four to five. For a one- to two-year-old child, reduce the dosage by half. For an eight- to nine-year-old, increase the dosage by 50%.

Formula Rhyme

Jia and Zao, with Musk and Worm,

Unblock the channels, stir what's firm.

Chi Shao, Tao Ren, Hong Hua too—

Disperse the stasis, guide it through.

Lian Qiao, Chai Hu cleanse with care,

And Da Huang purges if bowels bear.

Hui Yan Zhu Yu Tang

Hui Yan Zhu Yu Tang (Expelling Blood Stasis from the Epiglottis Decoction)

This formula is used to treat cases where the patient begins choking when drinking water five to six days after the onset of pox.

Ingredients

Pin Yin	Latin Name	English Name	Amount (grams)
Tao Ren	Persicae Semen (mashed)	Peach Kernel (mashed)	15
Hong Hua	Carthemi Flos	Safflower	15
Gan Cao	Glycyrrhizae Radix	Licorice Root	9
Jie Geng	Platycodi Radix	Balloon Flower Root	9
Sheng Di Huang	Rehmanniae Radix	Rehmanniae Root	12

Pin Yin	Latin Name	English Name	Amount (grams)
Dang Gui	Angelicae Sinensis Radix	Angelica Root	6
Xuan Shen	Scrophulariae Radix	Figwort Root	3
Chai Hu	Bupleuri Radix	Hare's Ear Root	3
Zhi Ke	Aurantii Fructus	Bitter Orange	6
Chi Shao	Paeoniae Radix Rubra	Red Peony Root	6

Tao Ren (fried) 15g, Hong Hua 15g, Gan Cao 9g, Jie Geng 9g, Sheng Di Huang 12g, Dang Gui 6g, Xuan Shen 3g, Chai Hu 3g, Zhi Ke 6g, Chi Shao 6g

Preparation and Usage

Boil together with water and drink the decoction

This formula is designed for treating cases of choking on water occurring five to six days after the onset of pox. If the patient experiences both convulsions and choking after pox, it is due to Qi deficiency causing the epiglottis to fail to properly seal the airway. In such cases, treatment should follow the convulsion formula instead.

Formula Rhyme

Stasis in the throat's deep bend—

Tao Ren, Hong Hua help to mend.

Gan Cao, Jie Geng soothe the chest,

Sheng Di, Xuan Shen cool and rest.

Dang Gui, Chi Shao move the Blood,

Chai Hu, Zhi Qiao clear the flood.

When water chokes and Blood congeals—

This blend restores, the throat soon heals.

Zhi Xie Tiao Zhong Tang

Zhi Xie Tiao Zhong Tang (Diarrhea Stopping and the Middle Tonifying Decoction)

This formula is used to treat persistent diarrhea occurring six to seven days after the onset of pox, or even after ten days or more.

Ingredients

Pin Yin	Latin Name	English Name	Amount (grams)
Huang Qi	Astragali Radix	Astragalus Root	24
Dang Shen	Codonopsis Radix	Codonopsis	9
Gan Cao	Glycyrrhizae Radix	Licorice Root	9
Bai Zhu	Atractylodis Macrocephalae Rhizoma	White Atractylodes	9
Dang Gui	Angelicae Sinensis Radix	Angelica Root	6
Bai Shao	Paeoniae Radix Alba	White Peony Root	6
Chuan Xiong	Chuanxiong Rhizoma	Cnidium	3
Hong Hua	Carthemi Flos	Safflower	9

Pin Yin	Latin Name	English Name	Amount (grams)
(Zhi) Fu Zi	Aconiti Radix Lateralis Preparata	Aconite Accessory Root	3
Liang Jiang	Rhizoma Alpiniae Officinarum	Galanga	1.5
Guan Gui (Rou Gui)	Cortex Cinnamomi	Cinnamon Bark	1.5

Huang Qi 24g, Dang Shen 9g, Gan Cao 6g, Bai Zhu 6g, Dang Gui 6g, Bai Shao 6g, Chuan Xiong 3g, Hong Hua 9g, Fu Zi (Zhi) 3g, Liang Jiang 1.5g, Guan Gui (no bark) 1.5g

Preparation and Usage

Boil together with water and drink the decoction

"This formula is designed for diarrhea occurring six to seven days after the onset of pox. It is also effective in cases where diarrhea accompanies convulsions following pox. However, it is not intended for treating diarrhea that appears at the early stage of pox eruption.

Formula Rhyme

Shen, Cao, and Qi to lift and tone,

Zhu, Gui, Shao Yao guide alone.

Hong Hua, Chuan Xiong move with care,

Fu Zi, Liang Jiang, Gui—just a share.

For Qi-deficient loose bowels you see,

This warming blend works steadily.

Bao Yuan Hua Zhi Tang

Bao Yuan Hua Zhi Tang (Vitality Protecting and Stagnation Clearing Decoction)

This formula is for treating dysentery occurring five to six days after the onset of pox. It is effective whether the dysenteric discharge is white, red, or a mixture of both.

Ingredients

Pin Yin	Latin Name	English Name	Amount (grams)
Huang Qi	Astragali Radix	Astragalus Root	30
Hua Shi	Talcum	Talc	30

Huang Qi 30g, Hua Shi (powder) 30g

Preparation and Usage

Biol Huang Qi (Astragali Radix / Astragalus Root) with water and add Hua Shi (Talcum / Talc) powder to the Huang Qi (Astragali Radix / Astragalus Root) decoction to drink. If taken at night, adding 1.5g of sugar is even better.

This formula is based on my clinical experience. It is effective not only for dysentery caused by pediatric pox but also shows remarkable results for both acute and chronic dysentery in adults. For acute adult dysentery, use 45 grams of Hua Shi (Talcum) and 30 grams of white sugar, Huang Qi (Astragalus Root) is not necessary. For chronic dysentery in adults, Huang Qi should be added, while Hua Shi remains at 45 grams."

Formula Rhyme

Boil one liang of Huang Qi to tonify Qi.

Add one liang of powdered Hua Shi to clear damp heat.

Together they treat dysentery with gentle might.

The bowels calm, and Qi stays bright.

Zhu Yang Zhi Yang Tang

Zhu Yang Zhi Yang Tang (Yang Supporting and Itch Stopping Decoction)

This formula is used to treat incessant itching after six to seven days of pox, where scratching breaks the skin without causing bleeding. It is also effective for treating loss of voice or hoarseness.

This formula is for treating severe itching that occurs six to seven days after the onset of pox, where scratching breaks the skin without causing bleeding. It is not intended for the mild itching that may occur during the first one to two days of pox.

Ingredients

Pin Yin	Latin Name	English Name	Amount (grams)
Huang Qi	Astragali Radix	Astragalus Root	30
Tao Ren	Persicae Semen (mashed)	Peach Kernel (mashed)	6
Hong Hua	Carthemi Flos	Safflower	6
Zao Jiao Ci	Spina Gleditsiae	Chinese Honey Locust Spine	3
Chi Shao	Paeoniae Radix Rubra	Red Peony Root	3
Chuan Shan Jia	Squama Manitis	Pangolin Scales	3

Huang Qi 30g, Tao Ren (mashed) 6g, Hong Hua 6g, Zao Ci 3g, Chi Shao 3g, Shan Jia (fried) 3g

Formula Rhyme

Huang Qi, Tao Ren, and Hong Hua move with might,

Zao Ci, Chi Shao, Shan Jia set things right.

For hoarse voice or lost sound, the path is one—

When Qi can't move, and surface strength is gone.

Zu Wei He Rong Tang

Zu Wei He Rong Tang (Qi (energy) Strengthening and Blood Moderating Decoction)

This formula is used to treat convulsions following pox, including symptoms such as eyes rolled upward and fixed, neck and spine arched backward, clenched jaw, continuous drooling, unconsciousness, widespread ulceration, and persistent discharge of pus.

Pin Yin	Latin Name	English Name	Amount (grams)
Huang Qi	Astragali Radix	Astragalus Root	30
Gan Cao	Glycyrrhizae Radix	Licorice Root	6

Volume 2

Pin Yin	Latin Name	English Name	Amount (grams)
Bai Zhu	Atractylodis Macrocephalae Rhizoma	White Atractylodes	6
Dang Shen	Codonopsis Radix	Codonopsis	9
Bai Shao	Paeoniae Radix Alba	White Peony Root	6
Dang Gui	Angelicae Sinensis Radix	Angelica Root	6
Suan Zao Ren	Ziziphi Spinosae Semen	Sour Jujube Seed	6
Tao Ren	Persicae Semen (mashed)	Peach Kernel (mashed)	3
Hong Hua	Carthemi Flos	Safflower	3

Huang Qi 30g, Gan Cao 6g, Bai Zhu 6g, Dang Shen 9g, Bai Shao 6g, Dang Gui 3g, Zao Ren 6g, Tao Ren (mashed) 4.5g, Hong Hua 4.5g

Preparation and Usage

Boil them with water and drink the decoction

This formula is specifically designed to treat convulsions and widespread ulceration following pox. For convulsions caused by Qi deficiency after Cold Damage, epidemic illness, miscellaneous syndromes, or prolonged illness, refer to the specialized formulas in the Convulsion chapter.

Formula Rhyme

Huang Qi, Gan Cao, Bai Zhu restore,

Shen, Shao, Gui, Zao, Tao, Hong support more.

Convulsions aren't Wind, the old view is flawed—

Reviving Yang with this brings life back to accord.

On Shao Fu Zhu Yu Tang

On Shao Fu Zhu Yu Tang (Expelling Blood Stasis from the Lower Abdomen Decoction)

This formula treats lower abdominal masses with or without pain, lower abdominal fullness and distension, as well as back soreness and bloating at the onset of menstruation. It is also effective for cases where menstruation occurs three to five times a month, repeatedly starting and stopping, with blood that is purple, black, or contains clots; as well as for menorrhagia, abnormal uterine bleeding accompanied by lower abdominal pain, or pink discharge with leukorrhea. All of these can be treated with this formula, and its effectiveness is beyond full description.

Even more remarkable, this formula produces near-miraculous results in treating infertility. Begin taking the medicine on the first day of menstruation and continue for five consecutive doses. Conception is almost certain within four months.

To conceive a son, the sum of the husband's and wife's ages and the month of conception must result in an odd number. For example: if one partner is an odd age and the other even, choose an even-numbered lunar month to conceive a son; if both are odd or both are even, choose an odd-numbered month.

Note that the 'month' should not be calculated by the lunar calendar's first day, but by the solar term (节气) marking the start of that lunar month. Conception may sometimes occur

135

as late as the twentieth day, so recording the exact date is important.

If the timing is off and a daughter is born, do not doubt the efficacy of the method. I have used this formula personally and have more successful cases than I can count on my fingers.

In the Guiwei year of the Daoguang era (1823), Mr. Suna, a sixty-year-old official with the Zhili Municipal Administration, was deeply troubled by not having a son. He consulted me, and I assured him, "This matter is easily resolved." I instructed his wife to begin taking this prescription in June, five doses per month. She conceived in September and gave birth to a son on June 22 of the following year, in the Jiashen year. That son is now seven years old.

This prescription also possesses a remarkable ability to turn danger into safety. Some pregnant women, though strong and full of vital Qi, eating well and showing no signs of physical damage, inexplicably miscarry around the third month. Many suffer repeated miscarriages over several pregnancies. Yet most medical texts still focus on nourishing Yin and Blood, strengthening the Spleen and Stomach, and calming or stabilizing the fetus, while truly effective formulas are rare.

They fail to realize that retained blood stasis in the uterus takes up space. As the fetus continues to grow around the third month, the womb cannot accommodate it. The fetal sac becomes compressed and diseased, preventing blood from nourishing the fetus. The blood instead exits from the side, resulting in early signs of bleeding and eventual miscarriage.

Since blood cannot enter the fetal sac, the fetus receives no nourishment and is therefore lost to miscarriage. For those who have previously miscarried around the third month, or have suffered three to five consecutive miscarriages, and are now pregnant again, taking three to five doses (or even seven to eight doses) of this prescription around the second month of pregnancy can help. It will thoroughly eliminate the blood stasis in the uterus, creating space for the fetus to grow. This ensures the pregnancy will continue without incident.

If a miscarriage has already occurred, taking three to five doses of this formula before conceiving again will ensure a stable and healthy pregnancy. This prescription is truly excellent, curing illness, enabling conception, ensuring a healthy male birth, and protecting the fetus. It is, in every way, a perfect formula.

Shao Fu Zhu Yu Tang

Shao Fu Zhu Yu Tang (Expelling Blood Stasis from the Lower Abdomen Decoction)

Ingredients

Pin Yin	Latin Name	English Name	Amount (grams)
Xiao Hui Xiang	Foeniculi Fructus	Fennel Seed	7 pieces
Gan Jiang	Zingiberis Rhizoma	Dried Ginger	0.6
Yan Hu Suo (Yuan Hu)	Rhizoma Corydalis	Corydalis	3
Mo Yao	Myrrha	Myrrh	6
Dang Gui	Angelicae Sinensis Radix	Chinese Angelica Root	9
Chuan Xiong	Chuanxiong Rhizoma	Cnidium	6
Guan Gui (Rou Gui)	Cortex Cinnamomi	Cinnamon Bark	3
Chi Shao	Paeoniae Radix Rubra	Red Peony Root	6

Pin Yin	Latin Name	English Name	Amount (grams)
Pu Huang	Typhae Pollen	Cattail Pollen	9
Wu Ling Zhi	Faeces Trogopterori	Pteropus, Trogopterus	6

Xiao hui Xiang (fried) 7 (counts), Gan Jiang (fried) 0.6g, Yuan Hu 3g, Mo Yao (fried) 6g, Dang Gui 9g, Chuan Xiong 6g, Guan Gui 3g, Chi Shao 6g, Pu Huang (raw) 9g, Ling Zhi (fried) 6g

Preparation and Usage

Boil together with water and drink the decoction three times a day

Formula Rhyme

Hui Xiang and dry-fried Jiang warm the womb,

Yuan Hu, Mo Yao, Xiong, and Dang Gui resume.

Pu Huang, Ling Zhi, Chi Shao, Gui combine—

To move Blood and calm the fetus fine.

On Pregnancy, Labor and Retained Placenta

On Pregnancy (with note on difficult labor and retained placenta)

Ancient theories claimed that the fetus in the uterus is nourished in monthly turns by different meridians: the Liver meridian in the first month, the Gallbladder in the second, the Heart in the third, the Triple Burner in the fourth, the Spleen in the fifth, the Stomach in the sixth, the Lung in the seventh, the Large Intestine in the eighth, and the Kidney in the ninth. According to this logic, when the fetus reaches the second month, the Liver would naturally "hand over" to the Gallbladder to take over nourishment. But this kind of theory is both emotionless and irrational.

The reality is simple: the fetus grows entirely by relying on the mother's blood. This one sentence explains everything, why make up theories just to chase fame and mislead others?

Another example is the so-called "baby crying theory," which claims that the fetus sucks blood by holding the umbilical cord in its mouth. But I ask, when the embryo first forms and has no mouth, what is it using to suck blood? If people do not understand this clearly, why not go back to study actual pregnant women, consult midwives, and gather real evidence? Only then should they write books. That way, they won't end up being ridiculed by future generations.

In the first month of pregnancy, there is no placenta. It begins to form after one month and develops during the second month. Once the placenta is fully formed, the fetus is already positioned. The placenta has two parts: a thicker section with two layers, which stores blood, and a thinner section with a single layer, which houses the fetus. Between these two sections, a narrow channel forms, the umbilical cord, which connects downward to the fetus's navel.

The mother's blood enters the thick, blood-filled part of the placenta, then flows into the umbilical cord to nourish the internal organs and limbs. The fetus develops as a whole, not in a sequence where some organs grow before others.

If miscarriage occurs within one month, there is no visible placenta. A two-month miscarriage will have a placenta shaped like a scale weight, small at the top, wider at the base, and no longer than three fingers. By three months, the fetus has formed eyes, ears, nose, and mouth, though the hands and feet remain in a clenched form, with fingers not yet distinct.

When full term approaches, the fetus pushes through the placenta, turns head-down, and is born. The placenta follows the baby, and the blood it contains is expelled along with it. This describes the true process of fetal development.

The most critical concern is difficult labor (dystocia). In the past, there was a traditional formula called *Kai Gu San* (Pelvis-Opening Powder). Some found it effective, while others did not. This formula focused primarily on promoting blood circulation and loosening the pelvic bones but overlooked exhaustion from physical exertion.

Whenever I use *Kai Gu San*, I always combine it with a large dose of *Huang Qi* (Astragali Radix / Astragalus Root). In every case, the baby is delivered within one hour.

As for retained placenta, there was an old remedy called *Mo Jie San* (Myrrh and Dragon's Blood Powder). When I first used it, results were mixed, effective for some, ineffective for others. Later, I began doubling the dosage, and the placenta would be expelled immediately.

The choice of herbs is certainly important, but even more important is the dosage.

Traditional Kai Gu San

Traditional Kai Gu San (Traditional Pelvis Opening Powder)

To treat dystocia.

Ingredients

Pin Yin	Latin Name	English Name	Amount (grams)
Huang Qi	Astragali Radix	Astragalus Root	120
Dang Gui	Angelicae Sinensis Radix	Angelica Root	30
Chuan Xiong	Chuanxiong Rhizoma	Cnidium	15

Pin Yin	Latin Name	English Name	Amount (grams)
Gui Ban	Testudinis Plastrum	Tortoise Plastron	24
Xue Yu	Crinis Carbonisatus	Charred Human Hair	A small bundle of hair

Dang Gui 30g, Chuan Xiong 15g, Gui Ban 24g, Xue Yu (ash) a small bundle

Adding Huang Qi (Astragali Radix / Astragalus Root) (raw) 120g

Preparation and Usage

Boil together with water and drink the decoction

Traditional Mo Jie San

Traditional Mo Jie San (Traditional Myrrh and Dragon Blood Powder)

For retained placenta. This formula is designed to treat retained placenta, when the placenta does not come out after childbirth.

Ingredients

Pin Yin	Latin Name	English Name	Amount (grams)
Mo Yao	Myrrha	Myrrh	9
Xue Jie	Calamus Draco	Dragon Blood	9

Mo Yao 9g, Xue Jie 9g

Preparation and Usage: Make powder, mix them and drink with boiled hot water

Huang Qi Tao Hong Tang

Huang Qi Tao Hong Tang (Astragalus, Peach Kernel and Safflower Decoction)

To Treat Postpartum Convulsions. This formula is used to treat convulsions after childbirth, characterized by dazed or fixed eyes, drooling from the mouth, reverse arching of the neck and back, and loss of consciousness.

Ingredients

Pin Yin	Latin Name	English Name	Amount (grams)
Huang Qi	Astragali Radix	Astragalus Root	240
Tao Ren	Persicae Semen (mashed)	Peach Kernel (mashed)	9
Hong Hua	Carthemi Flos	Safflower	6

Huang Qi (raw) 240g, Tao Ren (mashed) 9g, Hong Hua 6g

Preparation and Usage: Boil together with water and drink the decoction

Among all gynecology books, *Ji Yin Gang Mu* (*The Essential Compendium of Assisting Women*) is the best. The *Golden Mirror of Medicine* (*Yi Zong Jin Jian*) selected its key formulas and theories and adapted them into mnemonic verses for easier reading and memorization. However, for the condition of convulsions, the formulas provided were ineffective, this I have now supplemented with effective remedies.

Traditional Xia Yu Xue Tang

Traditional Xia Yu Xue Tang (Traditional Blood Stasis Purging Decoction)

To treat blood bulge. How can it be identified? The abdominal skin shows distended blue veins, and the belly is visibly enlarged, this indicates a case of Blood Buldge.

Ingredients

Pin Yin	Latin Name	English Name	Amount (grams)
Tao Ren	Persicae Semen (mashed)	Peach Kernel (mashed)	9
Da Huang	Rhei Radix Et Rhizoma	Rhubarb Root	1.5
Tu Bie Chong	Eupolyphaga Sinensis	Wingless Cockroach	3 whole
Gan Sui	Radix Euphorbiae Kansui	Kan-Sui Root, Euphorbia	1.5 or 2.4

Tao Ren 24g, Da Huang 1.5g, Tu Bie Chong 3 counts, Gan Sui (powder to drink) 1.5g (or 2.4g)

Preparation and Usage

Boil together with water except Gan Sui powder which is to be taken with the decoction.

Need to take it with aforementioned Ge Xia Zhu Yu Tang (Expelling Stasis from Under the Diaphragm Decoction) in turns to be more effective.

Chou Hu Lu Jiu (Gourd Wine)

To treat enlarged belly with swelling all over the body

Dry out a calabash gourd by self-draining, then roast it and grind into powder. Take 9 grams mixed with yellow wine. If the gourd is large, fill it with yellow wine and simmer for one hour, then drink the wine, this method is quite effective. The idea is to harness the gourd's natural draining property.

Mi Cong Zhu Dan Tang

Mi Cong Zhu Dan Tang (Honey, Green Onion and Pig Bile Decoction)

To treat swelling all over the body without enlarged belly

Bile from one whole Pig gallbladder, Honey 120g, mix these two ingredients

Green Onion head (one cun of the white) 4 pieces, Yellow Wine 250g, heat the green onion whites with yellow wine for two to three boils.

Then pour the boiled wine into the mix of honey and bile. Take it and the effect is immediate

Ci Wei Pi San (Hedgehog Skin Powder)

To treat spermatorrhea, whether accompanied by dreams or not, this remedy is effective for both deficiency and excess patterns.

Use one hedgehog skin, roast it on a clay tile until dry, then grind it into powder. Take the powder with yellow wine in the morning.

It is truly effective, though unpalatable.

Xiao Hui Xiang Jiu (Fennel Seeds Wine)

To treat Chyluria (urine with White Turbid), commonly known as Deceiving White (Pian Bai), also known as gonorrhoeae. This condition arises from wind-cold invasion of the seminal pathway. Other decoctions have proven ineffective in treating it.

Xiao Hui Xiang (Foeniculi Fructus / Fennel Seed), 30 grams, dry-fried until yellow and ground into coarse powder.

Boil 250 grams of yellow wine, then pour it over the powder. Let it steep for 15 minutes, strain out the residue, and drink the wine.

On Blood Stasis in Bi Syndrome

All shoulder pain, arm pain, lower back pain, leg pain, or generalized body aches are classified as Bi Syndrome.

When it's clearly caused by wind-cold, yet warming and dispersing formulas fail to resolve it;

When it's clearly due to damp-heat, yet draining dampness and clearing heat proves ineffective;

And when the condition persists, leading to muscle wasting, it's then assumed to be a case of Yin deficiency, so Yin-nourishing herbs are given, still without result.

At that point, people often say:

"If the illness lies in the superficial layers, skin and vessels, it's easy to treat;

If it lies deep within the sinews and bones, it's difficult to cure."

But they fail to consider where exactly the wind-cold or damp-heat has entered.

- If the pathogen enters the Qi (energy) channels, the pain will wander and shift.

- If it enters the blood vessels, the pain will stay fixed in one spot.

- And if there is bodily weakness, it is the result of the illness, not the original cause of it.

If one keeps nourishing Yin without addressing the invading pathogen, where is that external evil supposed to go?

If one only tries to dispel wind-cold or drain damp-heat, while the blood has already congealed, it still won't flow.

Think of water exposed to wind and cold, it freezes into ice.

By the time it becomes ice, the wind and cold are already gone.

If you understand this, treating Bi Syndrome is not difficult.

Ancient formulas offer many useful options.

But if none are effective, use this formula:

Shen Tong Zhu Yu Tang

Shen Tong Zhu Yu Tang (Expelling Blood Stasis for Body Ache Decoction)

Ingredients

Pin Yin	Latin Name	English Name	Amount (grams)
Qin Jiao	Gentianae Macrophyllae Radix	Gentiana Macrophylla Root	3
Chuan Xiong	Chuanxiong Rhizoma	Cnidium	6

Pin Yin	Latin Name	English Name	Amount (grams)
Tao Ren	Persicae Semen (mashed)	Peach Kernel (mashed)	9
Hong Hua	Carthemi Flos	Safflower	9
Gan Cao	Glycyrrhizae Radix	Licorice Root	6
Qiang Huo	Platycodi Radix	Balloon Flower Root	3
Mo Yao	Myrrha	Myrrh	6
Dang Gui	Angelicae Sinensis Radix	Angelica Root	9
Wu Ling Zhi	Faeces Trogopterori	Pteropus, Trogopterus	6
Xiang Fu	Cyperi Rhizoma	Cyperus	3
Niu Xi	Cyathulae Radix	Cyathula Root	9

Pin Yin	Latin Name	English Name	Amount (grams)
Di Long	Pheretima	Earthworm	6

Qin Jiao 3g, Chuan Xiong 6g, Tao Ren 9g, Hong Hua 9g, Gan Cao 6g, Qiang Huo 3g, Mo Yao 6g, Dang Gui 9g, Ling Zhi (fried) 6g, Xiang Fu 3g, Niu Xi 9g, Di Long 6g

Preparation and Usage

If there is a slight fever, add Cang Zhu (Atractylodis Rhizome) and Huang Bai (Phellodendron Bark).

If the patient is weak, consider adding 30 to 60 grams of Huang Qi (Astragalus Root).

Formula Rhyme

Niu Xi, Di Long, Qiang Huo ease pain,

Qin Jiao, Xiang Fu, Gui and Xiong remain.

Huang Qi, Cang Zhu, Huang Bai adjust if desired,

Wu Ling, Tao, Mo, and Hong are always required.

Nao Sha Wan (Sal Ammoniac Pill)

This formula treats scrofula and "rat sores" (deep suppurative nodules) that spread across the neck and chest, rupturing and discharging pus. It consistently produces rapid and effective results.

Ingredients

Pin Yin	Latin Name	English Name	Amount (grams)
Nao Sha	Sal Ammoniacus	Sal Ammoniac	6
Zao Jiao Zi	Spina Gleditsiae	Chinese Honey Locust Spine	100 counts

Ingredients and Preparation:

Nao Sha (Sal Ammoniac / Sal Ammoniacus), finely powdered – 6 grams

Zao Jiao Seeds (Spina Gleditsiae / Chinese Honey Locust Seeds) – 100 seeds

Aged Vinegar – 500 grams

Soak the Nao Sha and Zao Jiao Seeds in the vinegar for three days. Then transfer the mixture into a clay pot and simmer until nearly dry. Stir the remaining Nao Sha from the bottom of the pot into the partially dried Zao Jiao Seeds. Allow the mixture to dry naturally, or bake it gently over low heat, or warm it on a stove surface until fully dry.

Usage:

Chew 5 to 8 seeds each night, or take twice daily (morning and night), followed by warm boiled water.

Because the dried seeds can be very hard, it is also acceptable to grind them into powder for ingestion.

There are two types of Nao Sha (Sal Ammoniac / Sal Ammoniacus) used in this formula, red and white. I personally use the red variety. I am uncertain about the efficacy of the white one.

The red Nao Sha is obtained from a cave located in the northern mountains of Kuche (Kuqa). In summer, flames erupt from within the cave, making it impossible for anyone to approach. But in winter, the local Hui people enter the cave, completely unclothed, to retrieve it.

The *Materia Medica* claims that Nao Sha is produced by boiling salt brine from the Western Regions, likely referring to India or Tibet, but this is incorrect.

Dian Kuang Meng Xing Tang

Dian Kuang Meng Xing Tang (Mania Stopping Decoction)

Mania disorder is marked by uncontrollable episodes of crying or laughing, cursing, yelling, or singing, along with a loss of awareness of intimacy or social boundaries, and many other erratic behaviors. The root cause lies in the stagnation of Qi and blood, which prevents the Qi of the brain from properly connecting with that of the internal organs, much like being trapped in a dreamlike state.

Ingredients

Pin Yin	Latin Name	English Name	Amount (grams)
Tao Ren	Persicae Semen (mashed)	Peach Kernel (mashed)	24
Chai Hu	Bupleuri Radix	Hare's Ear Root	9
Xiang Fu	Cyperi Rhizoma	Cyperus	6
Chuan Mu Tong	Caulis Clematidis Armandii	Armand Clematis Stem, Anemone Clematis Stem	9
Chi Shao	Paeoniae Radix Rubra	Red Peony Root	9
Ban Xia	Pinelliae Rhizoma	Pinellia	6

Pin Yin	Latin Name	English Name	Amount (grams)
Da Fu Pi	Arecae Pericarpium	Magnetite	9
Qing Pi	Citri Reticulatae Viride Pericarpium	Immature Tangerine Peel	6
Chen Pi	Citri Reticulatae Pericarpium	Tangerine Peel	9
San Bai Pi	Mori Cortex	Mulberry Root Bark	12
Zi Su Zi	Perillae Fructus	Perilla Fruit	12
Gan Cao	Glycyrrhizae Radix	Licorice Root	15

Tao Ren 24g, Chai Hu 9g, Xiang Fu 6g, Mu Tong 9g, Chi Shao 9g, Ban Xia 6g, Fu Pi 9g, Qing Pi 6g, Chen Pi 9g, Sang Pi 12g, Su Zi (mashed) 12g, Gan Cao 15g

Preparation and Usage: Boil them together with water and drink the decoction

Formula Rhyme

Tao Ren, Chi Shao move Blood with care,

Xiang Fu, Chai Hu, Mu Tong clear the air.

Qing Pi, Ban Xia, Chen Pi, Fu Pi,

Sang Pi, Su Zi, double Gan Cao to repair.

Long Ma Zi Lai Dan

Long Ma Zi Lai Dan (Earthworm and Nux-vomica Seeds Pill)

Ingredients

Pin Yin	Latin Name	English Name	Amount (grams)
Ma Qian Zi	Semen Strychni	Nux-Vomica Seeds	240
Di Long	Pheretima	Earthworm	8 whole pieces

Ma Qian Zi (Semen Strychni) – 240g, Di Long (Pheretima / Earthworm) – 8 pieces (cleaned, baked, and ground into powder), Sesame Oil – 500g.

Preparation and Usage

Heat the sesame oil in a pot until it reaches a full boil. Add the Ma Qian Zi and fry until you hear a faint crackling sound. Remove one seed and cut it in half, when the interior shows a purplish-red hue, the degree of frying is appropriate. Grind the Ma Qian Zi into fine powder and mix thoroughly with the pre-prepared Di Long powder. Combine and knead the mixture into pills about the size of a mung bean.

Take 3 to 4 *fen* (approximately 1 gram) per dose at bedtime, with warm saltwater as a delivery medium. For children aged 5 to 6, reduce to 2 *fen* (about 0.5 grams) per dose and administer with brown sugar water.

If not made into pills, the powdered form can also be taken directly. For individuals who follow a vegetarian diet, the Di Long may be omitted.

To treat epilepsy, commonly referred to as *"Lamb Wind"* (羊羔风), begin by taking one dose of Huang Qi Chi Feng Tang (*Astragalus, Red Peony, and Siler Decoction*) each evening, followed by one dose of this pill at bedtime.

Continue both the decoction and the pill for one month. After that, discontinue the decoction and take only the pill. With long-term use, the condition will gradually resolve on its own. Once recovered, continue taking the pill for an additional one to two years to ensure complete eradication of the root cause.

The explanation of this condition can be found in the earlier section titled *"On the Brain."*

Huang Qi Chi Feng Tang

Huang Qi Chi Feng Tang (Astragalus, Red Peony and Siler Decoction)

Ingredients

Pin Yin	Latin Name	English Name	Amount (grams)
Huang Qi	Astragali Radix	Astragalus Root	60
Chi Shao	Paeoniae Radix Rubra	Red Peony Root	3
Fang Feng	Saposhnikoviae Radix	Siler	3

Huang Qi (raw) 60g, Chi Shao 3g, Fang Feng 3g

Preparation and Usage

Boil them together with water and drink the decoction. Half dose for children.

To treat leg paralysis, the dosage should be doubled. Continue taking the formula until the leg can move on its own, at that point, stop; do not exceed the required amount.

This formula is also effective for treating all types of sores, a wide range of illnesses, and general weakness following illness. Even when taken in the absence of disease, it does not cause harm and may help prevent illness.

In truth, the remarkable effects of this formula could not be fully described even in multiple essays. Its effectiveness across such a wide range of conditions lies in its ability to unblock the flow of Qi throughout the entire body and activate the blood, eliminating stasis. When Qi flows freely and blood circulates smoothly, how could illness possibly remain?

Huang Qi Fang Feng Tang

Huang Qi Fang Feng Tang (Astragalus and Siler Decoction)

To treat rectal prolapse, this formula has shown remarkable effectiveness, even in cases with a history of eight or ten years.

Pin Yin	Latin Name	English Name	Amount (grams)
Huang Qi	Astragali Radix	Astragalus Root	120

Pin Yin	Latin Name	English Name	Amount (grams)
Fang Feng	Saposhnikoviae Radix	Siler	3

Huang Qi (raw) 120g, Fang Feng 3g

Preparation and Usage: Boil then together and drink the decoction. Half dose for children

Huang Qi Gan Cao Tang

Huang Qi Gan Cao Tang (Astragalus and Licorice Decoction)

To treat sharp pain in the penis during urination in the elderly, this remedy delivers immediate relief, regardless of how long the condition has persisted.

Ingredients

Pin Yin	Latin Name	English Name	Amount (grams)
Huang Qi	Astragali Radix	Astragalus Root	120

Pin Yin	Latin Name	English Name	Amount (grams)
Gan Cao	Glycyrrhizae Radix	Licorice Root	24

Huang Qi (raw) 120g, Gan Cao 24g

Preparation and Usage

Boil them together and drink the decoction. Two doses a day for severe conditions.

Mu Er San (Wood Ear Powder)

Effective for all types of ulcerated sores, this formula yields results beyond description. It should not be underestimated.

Mu Er (Auricularia auricula / Wood Ear mushroom) – 30g, baked and ground into fine powder.

White Sugar – 30g, mix evenly.

Add warm water to form a paste. Apply directly to the affected area and wrap with a bandage.

From a fundamental perspective, this formula shares the same underlying principle as using hedgehog skin to treat spermatorrhea and drained dried gourd to treat enlarged belly and swelling.

Only by understanding this underlying principle can one truly begin to learn medicine.

Yu Long Gao

Yu Long Gao (Jade Dragon Ointment, also called Sheng Yu Gao)

For injuries caused by falls or blows, this topical application is highly effective.

Ingredients

Pin Yin	Latin Name	English Name	Amount (grams)
Zhi Ma You		Same Oil	500
Bai Lian	Ampelopsis Radix	Ampelopsis	12
Sheng Ma	Cimicifugae Rhizoma	Bugbane Rhizome	12
Dang Gui	Angelicae Sinensis Radix	Angelica Root	12
Chuan Xiong	Chuanxiong Rhizoma	Cnidium	12

Pin Yin	Latin Name	English Name	Amount (grams)
Lian Qiao	Forsythiae Fructus	Forsythia Fruit	12
Jin Yin Hua	Lonicerae Flos	Honeysuckle Flower	12
Chuan Shan Jia	Squama Manitis	Pangolin Scales	12
Chuan Wu	Aconiti Radix Preparata	Sichuan Aconite Root	12
Xiang Pi	Corium Elephantis	Elephant Hide	12
Ru Xiang	Olibanum	Frankincense	1.5
Mo Yao	Myrrha	Myrrh	1.5
Qing Fen	Calomelas	Calomel	9
Bing Pian	Borneolum	Borneol	1
She Xiang	Moschus	Musk	1
Bai La	Cera Chinensis	Insect White Wax	60

Sesame oil 500g, Bai Lian, Sheng Ma, Dang Gui, Chuan Xiong, Lian Qiao, Yin Hua, Jia Pian, Chuan Wu and Xiang Pi 12g each, Ru Xiang (powder) 1.5g, Mo Yao (powder) 1.5g, Qing Fen (powder) 9g, Bing Pian 1g (3 Fen), She Xiang 1g (3 Fen), Bai La 60g

Preparation and Usage

Fry the first nine herbs in sesame oil until they turn golden and slightly charred. Strain out the dregs. While still warm but off the heat, stir in three packets of *Guan Fen* (official-grade calomel powder). Then add Ru Xiang, Mo Yao, Qing Fen, Bing Pian, and She Xiang. Mix thoroughly. Finally, add the white wax and stir until it melts and blends uniformly.

Spread the resulting paste onto cloth or gauze and apply as a medicated patch to the affected area.

Note:

If you omit the *Guan Fen*, the resulting ointment (called *Gao Zi Yao*) is especially effective for suppurating sores and ulcerated wounds. Its healing effects are said to be near miraculous.

Mu Er San (Wood Ear Powder) and Yu Long Gao (Jade Dragon Ointment) are highly reliable remedies for all types of ulcerated and suppurating sores. Their effectiveness is proven and should never be underestimated.

On Effective Formulas and Theoretical Errors

Distinguishing Effective Formulas from Theoretical Errors, On the Mistaken Theory that Blood Transforms into Sweat

My nephew, Zuoli, came to the capital to visit me. When he saw *The Viscera Map* I had drawn, he asked, "Uncle, in your illustration, the meridians are shown as Qi vessels, all originating from the General Protective Vessel and spreading throughout the body. This suggests that the meridians form one interconnected system, rather than each organ having two fixed meridians."

I thought to myself, if the ancients truly did not understand the meridians, then how did Zhang Zhongjing, in his *Treatise on Cold Damage*, establish 113 formulas and outline 397 therapeutic methods, all based on the symptomatic patterns of the six Foot meridians? So many of his prescriptions have proven effective. I don't quite understand the logic here.

I replied, "Look at the first chapter of his book and study it carefully. You'll understand why his formulas are effective despite flaws in his theoretical framework. That chapter explains how, when the Foot Taiyang Bladder Channel is invaded by cold, it results in headache, body aches, stiff neck, fever, chills, retching, and absence of sweating. The treatment prescribed is *Ma Huang Tang* (Ephedra Decoction). If similar symptoms appear but with sweating, it is considered a Wind-induced febrile condition and treated with *Gui Zhi Tang* (Cinnamon Twig Decoction).

The discussion centers on the Foot Taiyang channel, which governs the legs but does not connect to the hands. Yet Zhang Zhongjing speaks of disease transmission between channels, only among the six leg channels, with no mention of the six hand channels. This reveals a key inconsistency in the theory of meridian progression."

Look at the onset of Cold Damage: symptoms include headache, body aches, stiff neck, fever, and aversion to cold, but no one experiences only pain or chills in just the arms and hands. When treated with *Ma Huang Tang* (Ephedra Decoction), the entire body recovers; there is no case where only the arms and hands remain ill. Doesn't this clearly prove that while the prescription is effective, the meridian theory behind it is flawed?

If, before Zhang Zhongjing, someone had directly observed the internal organs and written clearly that all meridians are interconnected, then when Zhongjing wrote *On Cold Damage*, he would simply have said: "When external cold invades the body's meridians, use *Ma Huang Tang* to disperse the cold from the entire system." One sentence would have sufficed.

The theory that febrile illness with sweating is Wind Damage and should be treated with *Gui Zhi Tang* (Cinnamon Twig Decoction) is, in my observation, unconvincing. This formula, composed of only three herbs, *Gui Zhi* (Cinnamon Twig), *Bai Shao* (White Peony Root), and *Gan Cao* (Licorice Root), has never, to my knowledge, cured a single person. The reason *Gui Zhi Tang* fails is because the symptoms of headache, body aches, fever, and sweating do not reflect Wind Damage, but rather align with the Plague Disorders (*Wen Yi Bing*) described by Wu Youke.

He asked again: "When cold evil remains on the exterior of the body, we should naturally see symptoms like headache, body aches, fever, aversion to cold, and absence of sweat. But why is there already the interior symptom of vomiting at the very onset of cold damage, before the illness has progressed internally? Zhang Zhongjing authored *On Cold Damage*, and dozens of scholars, including Wang Shuhe, wrote commentaries on it, yet none of them explained why vomiting occurs during an exterior syndrome. I truly cannot understand this and humbly ask uncle to enlighten me."

I replied: "At first, I thought you merely had a scholarly interest in reading, but lacked the ability to truly practice medicine. Now, hearing your question, I see that you have a capacity for deeper reasoning. In the future, you will not need to fear causing harm through ignorance or negligence."

You asked why, when cold evil is on the exterior, there is the interior symptom of vomiting. Let me explain this to you in detail: Cold evil first enters through the pores, then penetrates the skin, from the skin into the minute collaterals (sun luo), then into the yang collaterals (yang luo), then into the main meridians. From the meridians it reaches the General Protective Vessel (wei zong guan), which traverses into the heart. From the heart, it ascends into the left and right Qi conduits, which in turn attack the left and right Qi gates near the throat, thereby inducing vomiting. This is the true reason why an exterior pattern can present with vomiting.

When Ma Huang Tang (Ephedra Decoction) is taken into the stomach, the liquid essence of the herbs flows out through the Fluid Gate, enters the fluid ducts, passes through the liver, and then enters the fine ducts within the spleen. From there, it seeps through the water pathways and is filtered into the bladder, eventually becoming urine. Meanwhile, the Qi of the medicine, its active therapeutic property, travels from the fluid ducts into the General Protective Vessel (Wei Zong Guan), from there into the meridians, then into the collateral vessels, from the collaterals into the minute collaterals, from the minute collaterals to the skin, and finally to the pores. The cold evil is expelled outward through the pores, resulting in sweating. As sweat is released, the pathogenic evil is carried out with it. Once the evil is dispersed through sweat, the vomiting ceases. This illustrates the full connectivity of the body's internal and external meridians and collaterals, and the mechanism by which Ma Huang Tang disperses external pathogens through the action of sweating.

He asked again: "Zhang Zhongjing said that symptoms such as eye pain, dry nose, and insomnia are exterior signs of the Foot Yangming Stomach meridian, and treated them with Ge Gen Tang (Kudzu Decoction). The formula contains both Ge Gen (Kudzu Root) and Ma Huang (Ephedra). I don't quite understand the rationale behind this."

I replied: "When cold evil enters the body from the exterior and invades the meridians, the upright Qi (Zheng Qi) transforms this cold into heat, this is what we call *evil heat*.

When evil heat ascends to attack the head, it disturbs the brain, resulting in insomnia. The visual system connects upward to the brain, and when evil heat enters the eyes from the brain, the eyes become painful. Likewise, the nose is connected to the brain, and the evil heat traveling there causes nasal dryness. These are clearly fire-like symptoms caused by ascending evil heat, not simply an exterior cold pattern of the Foot Yangming Stomach meridian.

The reason Ge Gen (Kudzu Root) is effective here is because it is a cool-dispersing herb, not a warm-dispersing one, as some might assume. As for Ma Huang (Ephedra), it is included to disperse the residual cold that remains on the exterior and has not yet transformed. This again demonstrates a case where the formula is effective, but the meridian theory behind it is mistaken."

He asked again: "Zhang Zhongjing discussed symptoms such as hypochondriac pain, deafness, bitter taste in the mouth, alternating chills and fever, and vomiting. He said this pattern lies halfway between the exterior and interior, the Shaoyang stage, and is a disorder of the Foot Shaoyang Gallbladder meridian, to be treated with *Xiao Chai Hu Tang* (Minor Bupleurum Decoction). His formula is remarkably effective. But when I reflect on this: if the illness is **not** in the Gallbladder meridian, why is the formula so effective? And if it **is** in the Gallbladder meridian, the gallbladder is located below the diaphragm, yet the pain manifests in the hypochondrium. This confuses me."

I replied: "Look at the viscera map, at the *Blood Chamber* (血府) located above the diaphragm, and you'll understand. The evil heat enters the Blood Chamber and assaults the blood there, resulting in pain in the hypochondriac region. As the evil moves inward to attack the blood, and the blood resists outward to defend, this dynamic tension creates alternating chills and fever. When the heat scorches the left and right *Qi valves*, Qi becomes obstructed and cannot ascend or descend freely, this leads to vomiting and bitterness in the mouth. When the evil heat rises further, it attacks the upper orifices, causing deafness and dizziness.

Chai Hu (Bupleurum) has the ability to clear heat from the Blood Chamber. Once the heat is dispersed, sweat comes out naturally, carrying the evil with it, thus the symptoms resolve swiftly. This, again, is a case where the formula is effective, but the meridian-based theory is incorrect.

As for the complex changes and developments of disease patterns, they ultimately do not go beyond the fundamental categories of *interior vs. exterior* and *deficiency vs. excess*. If you truly wish to understand Cold Damage illnesses, you must study Wu Youke's *Treatise on Pestilential Diseases*. Reading too few books will leave you prone to one-sided errors, leaning either too much toward cold or toward heat."

Last night, you asked in front of our guest: the ancients said that within the skin, sweat is blood, and once it emerges, it becomes sweat, that sweat is transformed from blood. You said you didn't understand this principle. I didn't explain it to you at the time, not because you spoke too much in front of the guest, but because the guest is still new to medicine and not yet an expert. That's why I chose not to answer in front of him.

The idea that sweat is transformed from blood was proposed by Danxi Zhu Zhenheng. Although Zhang Jingyue critiqued and refuted Zhu's theory, he was ultimately unable to clearly identify the true origin of sweat. The fundamental mistake made by the ancients lies in their failure to understand that Qi and blood travel through two distinct systems: Qi flows through vessels that connect to the skin and open via pores, hence sweat can be released. Blood flows through vessels that also reach the skin but have no pores, therefore, blood does not exit through the skin in the same way.

How can we be sure that blood vessels connect to the skin without pores? Observe skin ulcers that rupture and leak yellow fluid. These toxins come from the Qi vessels. The yellow fluid flows continuously, yet the skin remains unreddened. But if the toxin originates from the blood vessels, the skin will first turn red. When it ulcerates, what flows out is purulent blood. Likewise, in epidemic illnesses, eruptions, rashes, or childhood pox, though the skin appears red, there is no bleeding. Isn't this solid evidence that blood vessels, while reaching the skin, lack any pores?

My nephew Zuoli came to the capital and raised these questions during a casual conversation. At that time, the book had already been engraved, so I recorded this exchange at the end of the volume.

About the Translator

Dr. Forest Yin (尹明杰) is a Doctor of Acupuncture and Oriental Medicine (DAOM), licensed acupuncturist, herbalist, and professor of Traditional Chinese Medicine. He currently serves as a professor and doctoral advisor at the University of East West Medicine in California.

Dr. Yin earned his degree in Modern Physics from the University of Science and Technology of China (USTC) and previously held senior executive roles at leading global technology firms in Silicon Valley. Since his college years, he has devoted himself to the study and clinical practice of Chinese medicine and natural healing—integrating Eastern wisdom with modern science to support genuine health, spiritual insight, and mindful living.

He is the author of the Chinese philosophical and medical work *Healing Wisdom of a Sage* (《明医至言》) and the ten-book English series *The Medicine-Free, Illness-Free Series,* which introduces practical, science-informed natural therapies for everyday well-being.

This translation of *Medical Forest Error Corrections* reflects his commitment to preserving, clarifying, and transmitting the classical foundations of Chinese medicine to a wider global audience.

Medical Forest Error Corrections

For questions, feedback, or professional inquiries:

Info@ashihealing.com

www.ingramcontent.com/pod-product-compliance
Lightning Source LLC
Chambersburg PA
CBHW022317280326
41932CB00010B/1130